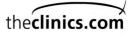

theclinics.com

VETERINARY CLINICS

OF NORTH AMERICA

Small Animal Practice

Pediatrics

GUEST EDITOR
Autumn P. Davidson, DVM, MS

May 2006 • Volume 36 • Number 3

SAUNDERS

An Imprint of Elsevier, Inc.
PHILADELPHIA   LONDON   TORONTO   MONTREAL   SYDNEY   TOKYO

W.B. SAUNDERS COMPANY
A Division of Elsevier Inc.

Elsevier, Inc., 1600 John F. Kennedy Blvd., Suite 1800, Philadelphia, PA 19103-2899

http://www.vetsmall.theclinics.com

VETERINARY CLINICS OF NORTH AMERICA:	**Volume 36, Number 3**
SMALL ANIMAL PRACTICE	**ISSN 0195-5616**
May 2006	**ISBN 1-4160-3583-4**

Editor: John Vassallo

The ideas and opinions expressed in *Veterinary Clinics of North America: Small Animal Practice* do not necessarily reflect those of the Publisher. The Publisher does not assume any responsibility for any injury and/or damage to persons or property arising out of or related to any use of the material contained in this periodical. The reader is advised to check the appropriate medical literature and the product information currently provided by the manufacturer of each drug to be administered to verify the dosage, the method and duration of administration, or contraindications. It is the responsibility of the treating physician or other health care professional, relying on independent experience and knowledge of the patient, to determine drug dosages and the best treatment for the patient. Mention of any product in this issue should not be construed as endorsement by the contributors, editors, or the Publisher of the product or manufacturers' claims.

Veterinary Clinics of North America: Small Animal Practice (ISSN 0195-5616) is published bimonthly (For Post Office use only: volume 36 issue 3 of 6) by W.B. Saunders, 360 Park Avenue South, New York, NY 10010-1710. Months of publication are January, March, May, July, September, and November. Business and Editorial Offices: 1600 John F. Kennedy Blvd., Suite 1800, Philadelphia, PA 19103-2899. Accounting and circulation offices: 6277 Sea Harbor Drive, Orlando, FL 32887-4800. Periodicals postage paid at New York, NY and additional mailing offices. Subscription prices are $170.00 per year for US individuals, $275.00 per year for US institutions, $85.00 per year for US students and residents, $225.00 per year for Canadian individuals, $345.00 per year for Canadian institutions, $235.00 per year for international individuals, $345.00 per year for international institutions and $115.00 per year for Canadian and foreign students/residents. To receive student/resident rate, orders must be accompanied by name of affiliated institution, date of term, and the *signature* of program/residency coordinator on institution letterhead. Orders will be billed at individual rate until proof of status is received. Foreign air speed delivery is included in all *Clinics* subscription prices. All prices are subject to change without notice. **POSTMASTER**: Send address changes to *Veterinary Clinics of North America: Small Animal Practice*, Elsevier Periodicals Customer Service, 6277 Sea Harbor Drive, Orlando, FL 32887-4800, USA; phone: 1-800-654-2452 [toll free number for US customers], or (+1)(407) 345-4000 [customers outside US]; fax: (+1)(407) 363-1354; email: usjcs@elsevier.com.

Veterinary Clinics of North America: Small Animal Practice is also published in Japanese by Gakusosha Company Ltd., 2-16-28 Nishikata, Bunkyo-ku, Tokyo 113, Japan.

Reprints: For copies of 100 or more, of articles in this publication, please contact the Commercial Reprints Department, Elsevier Inc., 360 Park Avenue South, New York, New York 10010-1710. Tel. (212) 633-3813 Fax: (212) 462-1935, email: reprints@elsevier.com

Veterinary Clinics of North America: Small Animal Practice is covered in *Current Contents/Agriculture, Biology and Environmental Sciences, Science Citation Index, ASCA, Index Medicus, Excerpta Medica, and BIOSIS.*

Printed in the United States of America.

ELSEVIER
SAUNDERS

VETERINARY CLINICS
SMALL ANIMAL PRACTICE

Pediatrics

GUEST EDITOR

AUTUMN P. DAVIDSON, DVM, MS, Diplomate, American College of Veterinary Internal Medicine; Clinical Professor, Department of Medicine and Epidemiology, School of Veterinary Medicine, Veterinary Medical Teaching Hospital Small Animal Clinic, University of California at Davis, Davis, California

CONTRIBUTORS

TOMAS W. BAKER, MS, Chief Ultrasonographer, Department of Surgery and Radiological Sciences, School of Veterinary Medicine, Veterinary Medical Teaching Hospital Small Animal Clinic, University of California at Davis, Davis, California

DANIKA L. BANNASCH, DVM, PhD, Chief, Genetics Service, Veterinary Medical Teaching Hospital and Assistant Professor, Department of Population Health and Reproduction, School of Veterinary Medicine, University of California at Davis, Davis, California

AUTUMN P. DAVIDSON, DVM, MS, Diplomate, American College of Veterinary Internal Medicine; Clinical Professor, Department of Medicine and Epidemiology, School of Veterinary Medicine, Veterinary Medical Teaching Hospital Small Animal Clinic, University of California at Davis, Davis, California

GINA M. DAVIS-WURZLER, DVM, Assistant Clinical Professor, Department of Veterinary Medicine and Epidemiology, School of Veterinary Medicine; Service Chief, Small Animal Outpatient Medicine, Veterinary Medical Teaching Hospital, University of California at Davis, Davis, California

DEBORAH S. GRECO, DVM, PhD, Diplomate, American College of Veterinary Internal Medicine; Staff Internist, The Animal Medical Center, New York, New York

SOPHIE A. GRUNDY, BVSc (Hons), MACVSc, Diplomate, American College of Veterinary Internal Medicine; Graduate Student Researcher, Department of Population Health and Reproduction, School of Veterinary Medicine, University of California at Davis, Davis, California

ANGELA M. HUGHES, DVM, Resident in Genetics, Veterinary Medical Teaching Hospital, School of Veterinary Medicine, University of California at Davis, Davis, California

JAMES A. LAVELY, DVM, Diplomate, American College of Veterinary Internal Medicine (Neurology); The Animal Care Center, Rohnert Park, California

KRISTIN A. MACDONALD, DVM, PhD, Diplomate, American College of Veterinary Internal Medicine (Cardiology); Veterinary Cardiologist, The Animal Care Center of Sonoma, Rohnert Park; Adjunct Faculty, Department of Surgical and Radiological Sciences, University of California at Davis, Davis, California

MICHAEL L. MAGNE, DVM, MS, Diplomate, American College of Veterinary Internal Medicine; Staff Internist, Animal Center of Sonoma County, Rohnert Park, California

TERRY NAGLE, BVSc, MACVSc, Diplomate, American College of Veterinary Dermatology; VCA–Sacramento Animal Medical Group, Carmichael, California

STEFANO ROMAGNOLI, DVM, MS, PhD, Diplomate, European College of Animal Reproduction; Department of Veterinary Clinical Sciences, University of Padua, Padua, Italy

DONALD H. SCHLAFER, DVM, MS, PhD, Diplomate, American College of Veterinary Pathologists; Diplomate, American College of Theriogenologists; Diplomate, American College of Veterinary Microbiologists; Department of Biomedical Sciences, Cornell University, Ithaca, New York

VETERINARY CLINICS
SMALL ANIMAL PRACTICE

Pediatrics

CONTENTS VOLUME 36 • NUMBER 3 • MAY 2006

Congenital heart disease (CHD) is defined as a morphologic defect of the heart or associated great vessels present at birth. Abnormalities are caused by alterations or arrests in particular phases of embryonic development of the fetal heart. The term *congenital* does not imply that the defect was inherited, and the defect may have occurred spontaneously or secondary to a drug or toxin. By studying families of animals with specific CHDs, many defects have also been shown to be heritable. Additionally, if the defect was caused by a spontaneous de novo mutation, that individual has the potential to transmit the mutation to offspring. The diagnosis of CHD is important not only to the health of the patient but to eliminate affected individuals from the breeding pool.

This article discusses some of the more common gastrointestinal problems encountered in pediatric patients. Topics include infectious and endoparasitic disorders, congenital esophageal and hepatic disorders, and acute or chronic intestinal diseases. Diagnostic criteria as well as treatment guidelines are presented.

Endocrine and metabolic disorders affecting puppies and kittens from birth until 6 months of age may manifest as clinical problems related to growth or to water metabolism (polydipsia and polyuria). Most commonly, endocrine and metabolic disorders affect growth of the animal, and puppies are often presented to the veterinarian for assessment of delayed or aberrant growth. Other endocrine disorders of small animals, such as juvenile-onset diabetes insipidus or diabetes mellitus, affect water metabolism, resulting in excessive thirst and urination and resultant difficulty in house-breaking.

Skin conditions of puppies and kittens are often infectious, such as ectoparasites or dermatophytosis. Hereditary and congenital skin problems are often detected at an early age. Young animals may be more prone to toxicity from medications, and labels should be read carefully for age limits. Husbandry factors, including nutrition, ectoparasites, temperature and humidity, cleaning products, and bedding, should be considered. Fleas are still a common problem despite recent improvements in flea control and can be debilitating in young animals because of blood loss.

Disorders of Sexual Differentiation in Puppies and Kittens: A Diagnostic and Clinical Approach

Stefano Romagnoli and Donald H. Schlafer

As in all domestic mammals, sexual differentiation in dogs and cats starts early in the embryonic period prenatally and continues into early postnatal life. The result of such a process is, however, not evident until after puberty, a time when the entire reproductive system undergoes significant changes. Normality of sexual differentiation is difficult to observe in neonates of small animals, with the only gender difference being a slightly longer anogenital distance in male (13–15 mm) versus female (7–8 mm) animals. Early diagnosis of deviations from normality can spare breeders the time and effort devoted to raising an animal that may turn out to be unsuitable for becoming part of the reproductive stock and may spare owners the concern for a pet whose health may be unnecessarily threatened by failing to remove a malformed reproductive system early in life. This article reviews the incidence, clinical and gross anatomic features, and diagnostic approaches that veterinarians can use to address inborn errors of the reproductive system of dogs and cats, highlighting those malformations that bear clinical relevance and may become manifest from birth until puberty.

Current Vaccination Strategies in Puppies and Kittens

Gina M. Davis-Wurzler

Motivation in writing this article stems from many things: a lack of time spent in the veterinary curriculum discussing vaccines, a growing concern (by the general public and the veterinary community) regarding adverse reactions associated with vaccines, and a desire to prevent a recurrence of preventable infectious diseases resulting from a fear-driven cessation of vaccine administration. The objectives of this article are to present a basic review of immunology as related to vaccines, to discuss general guidelines for pediatric vaccines in canine and feline patients, and to offer suggestions as to how we can most positively influence our patients' health from the first visit.

Pediatric Abdominal Ultrasonography

Tomas W. Baker and Autumn P. Davidson

Pediatric patients are commonly presented to the veterinarian because of signs referable to the abdominal cavity caused by congenital anomalies, dietary indiscretion, parasitic infestation, and infectious disease. Abdominal ultrasound provides valuable clinical information about the peritoneal cavity, great vessels, abdominal viscera, and lymph nodes, which is obtained in a noninvasive fashion and usually does not necessitate sedation or anesthesia. Ultrasonography thus greatly facilitates diagnostic evaluation of the pediatric patient. Ultrasound equipment already in place in many small animal veterinary clinics is appropriate for most pediatric cases.

GOAL STATEMENT

The goal of the *Veterinary Clinics of North America: Small Animal Practice* is to keep practicing veterinarians up to date with current clinical practice in small animal medicine by providing timely articles reviewing the state of the art in small animal care.

ACCREDITATION

The *Veterinary Clinics of North America: Small Animal Practice* offers continuing education credits, awarded by Cummings School of Veterinary Medicine at Tufts University, Office of Continuing Education.

Cummings School of Veterinary Medicine at Tufts University is a designated provider of continuing veterinary medical education. Veterinarians participating in this learning activity may earn up to 6 credits per issue up to a maximum of 36 credits per year. Credits awarded may not apply toward license renewal in all states. It is the responsibility of each participant to verify the requirements of their state licensing board.

Credit can be earned by reading the text material, taking the examination online at *http://www.theclinics.com/home/cme*, and completing the program evaluation. Following your completion of the test and program evaluation, and review of any and all incorrect answers, you may print your certificate.

TO ENROLL

To enroll in the *Veterinary Clinics of North America: Small Animal Practice* Continuing Veterinary Medical Education Program, call customer service at 1-800-654-2452 or sign up online at *http://www.theclinics.com/home/cme*. The CVME program is now available at a special introductory rate of $99.95 for a year's subscription.

VETERINARY CLINICS
SMALL ANIMAL PRACTICE

ELSEVIER
SAUNDERS

FORTHCOMING ISSUES

RECENT ISSUES

Vet Clin Small Anim 36 (2006) xi

VETERINARY CLINICS
SMALL ANIMAL PRACTICE

ELSEVIER
SAUNDERS

PREFACE

Pediatrics

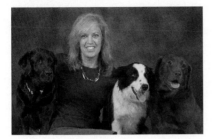

Autumn P. Davidson, DVM, MS

Guest Editor

P ediatric patients are great when they are healthy and presented for well puppy or kitten checks and routine vaccinations (but even those have become controversial). They are the darlings of practice, usually associated with happy and enthusiastic clients and serving to remind veterinary staff why clinical practice is fun and fulfilling.

When pediatric patients are sick, however, everything changes. Small and fragile, puppies and kittens defy routine diagnostics and therapeutics and are usually quite seriously ill when presented, demanding critical attention and informed intervention. Sick pediatric patients pose a special challenge to veterinarians and their staff. The reader should find every article in this issue helpful and insightful, as I did, when faced with pediatric cases.

Veterinary pediatrics has advanced into the subspecialties—exemplified in this issue—as our knowledge base has expanded. Great brains of extremely busy folk contributed to the effort to provide this informative resource for veterinary pediatric practice. I am most grateful to them, because the time spent on this issue was above and beyond busy clinical and academic practice in every instance.

Autumn P. Davidson, DVM, MS
Department of Medicine and Epidemiology
School of Veterinary Medicine
Veterinary Medical Teaching Hospital Small Animal Clinic
University of California at Davis
1 Shields Avenue
Davis, CA 95616, USA
E-mail address: apdavidson@ucdavis.edu

0195-5616/06/$ – see front matter
doi:10.1016/j.cvsm.2006.01.002

Vet Clin Small Anim 36 (2006) 443–459

VETERINARY CLINICS
SMALL ANIMAL PRACTICE

Clinically Relevant Physiology of the Neonate

Sophie A. Grundy, BVSc (Hons), MACVSc

Department of Population Health and Reproduction, School of Veterinary Medicine, University of California at Davis, Room 1114 Tupper Hall, 1 Shields Avenue, Davis, CA 95616, USA

Whant exactly is a neonate? Strictly speaking, the term *neonate* is derived from the Latin *natus* (to be born) and refers to a newborn during the first 4 weeks of life. The adoption of this term in canine and feline medicine is convenient, because weaning occurs approximately 4 weeks after birth; thus, for canine and feline patients, the neonatal period refers to that time between birth and weaning.

It is easy to be intimidated when presented with a sick neonate. Such patients are often not presented until late in the course of illness and weigh less than a kilogram. Venepuncture may be challenging, and standard physical examination techniques, such as auscultation and abdominal palpation, may be difficult. The key to demystifying canine and feline neonatal care is to cease considering such patients as miniature adults and, instead, to approach their management with an understanding and appreciation of their unique physiologic state and the transitions that take place during the neonatal period.

This article presents aspects of neonatal physiology in a body system approach that has clinical relevance so that the reader is able to appreciate the nuances of neonatal care and establish a routine approach for neonate evaluation, diagnostics, and treatment.

CARDIOVASCULAR SYSTEM

The cardiovascular system of the neonate undergoes dramatic alteration during the neonatal period as the fetomaternal circulation is lost and the neonatal heart assumes the role of maintaining circulatory homeostasis. This section focuses on the functional cardiovascular changes that occur in the neonate; for a discussion regarding pediatric cardiology, the reader is referred to the article by MacDonald in this issue. The neonate has a low-pressure, low-volume, and low peripheral resistance circulatory system [1,2]. It follows that to maintain peripheral perfusion, the neonate must maintain a higher heart rate, cardiac output, plasma volume, and central venous pressure as compared with the adult; thus, the neonatal

E-mail address: sagrundy@ucdavis.edu

0195-5616/06/$ – see front matter
doi:10.1016/j.cvsm.2005.12.002

circulation may be considered as a low-resistance–high-flow circuit [1,2]. During the neonatal period, systolic blood pressure in the canine neonate was noted to increase from 61 ± 5 mm Hg at birth to 139 ± 4 mm Hg at 4 weeks in a group of seven Beagle puppies [1]. This pressure change occurs in association with a decrease in heart rate from 204 ± 3 to 123 ± 6 beats per minute.

With respect to control of neonatal heart rate, studies suggest that in contrast to parasympathetic innervation of the heart, sympathetic innervation is incomplete [3]. Despite evidence of structural parasympathetic maturity, chronotropic responses in puppies at any given level of neural stimulus are less as compared with adult dogs, and before 14 days of age, there is minimal increase in heart rate in association with atropine administration, suggestive of a lack of vagal tone [3,4]. In kittens, vagal stimulation was found to have no effect on heart rate until 11 days of age [3]. These findings suggest a lack of full cardiac autonomic development during the neonatal period and help to explain why atropine is not effective in neonatal resuscitation (see below).

In comparison to alteration in heart rate attributable to autonomic stimulation, vasomotor tone, as indicated by the baroreceptor reflex, is functional and detected by 4 days of age [4]. Before 4 days of age, anoxia (10 minutes) results in profound bradycardia (45 beats per minute) and marked hypotension (systolic blood pressure of 23 mm Hg) [5]. This physiologic response is in direct contrast to that of the adult dog and is advantageous during parturition and the first few days of life. Remarkably, circulatory failure does not occur at such low systolic pressure in the neonate, and pups may be readily revived provided that the systolic blood pressure remains greater than 8 mm Hg [5]. Studies evaluating heart rate response to hypoxia (decrease in inspired oxygen from 21% to 17% fraction of inspired oxygen [FIO_2]) in a variety of newborn unanesthetized mammalian species failed to detect an alteration in heart rate [6].

Clinical Implications

One of the most important considerations of cardiovascular physiology in the neonate is that bradycardia is not vagally mediated and is indicative of hypoxemia in the fetus and during the first 4 days of life. Although the neonate seems to be able to resist circulatory failure to a greater extent than the adult animal during this time, it is far more appropriate to supplement oxygen than to give parasympatholytic agents, such as atropine, the administration of which only exacerbates cardiac hypoxemia via increasing oxygen demand in the face of hypoxemia.

Additionally, because of the incomplete maturity of the autonomic nervous system, the neonate is less able to respond to physiologic stresses. Care should be given to maintain the neonate environment so that demands on the cardiovascular system are minimal.

RESPIRATORY SYSTEM

Stimulation of the genital or umbilical region of the neonate induces reflex respiration in the first 3 days after birth and may be clinically used to stimulate respiration in the immediate postpartum period [7]. Normal respiratory rate in the neonate ranges from 10 to 18 breathes per minute at 1 day of age to 16 to 32 breathes per minute (comparable to that of an adult animal) by 1 week of age [4].

The mechanisms that control respiratory function in the newborn develop well before birth but require maturation in the postnatal period [8]. The neonate is susceptible to relative hypoxemia because of a large metabolic oxygen requirement and immaturity of carotid body chemoreceptors [8].

The biphasic ventilatory response to hypoxemia in the neonatal period has been well described: an initial increase in minute ventilation (increase in tidal volume and frequency), followed by a return to baseline [8]. Evaluation of the ventilatory response to hypoxia in the sleeping puppy revealed that ventilatory behavior is dependent on the stage of sleep [9]. During periods of prolonged hypoxia, minute ventilation is noted to decrease during quiet sleep but to increase during rapid eye movement (REM) sleep [9]. Although this phenomenon seems to illustrate metabolic and ventilatory uncoupling during REM sleep, the $PaCO_2$ does not rise and, in fact, decreases, suggestive of a decrease in metabolic rate to maintain metabolic and ventilatory coupling [8,9]. A similar ventilatory response to hypoxia was noted during the evaluation of anesthetized kittens; increased respiratory frequency and tidal volume were recorded [10].

The amount of work and pressure that is required by a neonate to maintain tidal breathing is increased as compared with that of an adult because of the high compliance of the chest wall [8]. Any respiratory disorder that shortens inspiratory duration has a greater potential to have a negative impact on gas exchange in the neonate [8].

Vagal cholinergic innervation of canine and feline airways is present and physiologically functional at birth [11]. Fisher and colleagues [11] demonstrated that electrical vagal stimulation resulted in an increased inspiratory resistance and decreased compliance in 1- to 14-day-old kittens and 3- to 14-day-old puppies that was prevented by the administration of atropine, suggesting muscarinic receptor activation. The effects of hypercapnia on pulmonary mechanics were evaluated in nine puppies 2 to 16 days of age; the hypercapnia resulted in increased inspiratory resistance that was eliminated with prior administration of atropine [12]. These findings suggest that that reflex bronchomotor tone and vagal efferent innervation to the airways are functional at birth [12]. In comparison, there is an inconsistent alteration in the pulmonary mechanical response (increased inspiratory resistance and decreased compliance) to hypoxia in canine and feline neonates; when present, there is a question as to whether it is attributable to a vagally mediated or direct response [12,13].

Clinical Implications

The neonate is susceptible to the development of hypoxemia or jeopardized ventilation and gas exchange because of the immaturity of chemoreceptor responses to hypoxia and chest wall construction. Although there are adaptations present to help compensate for this physiologic state, such as an extremely low circulatory failure pressure until 4 days of age, it is important to recognize that hypoxemia in the neonate may result in life-threatening sequelae, such as septic shock, because of bacterial translocation despite a lack of mucosal lesions [14].

It is vital that the environment be kept free of airway irritants. Adequate ambient temperature control should be maintained along with appropriate nutrition and oxygenation.

HEMATOPOIETIC SYSTEM

The general blood characteristics at varying ages for the cat and dog are well described [15]. At birth, the neonate red blood cell exhibits macrocytosis with corpuscle volume decreasing to that of the adult by 4 weeks of age as fetal red blood cells are replaced by adult red blood cells [15,16].

The hematocrit of the neonate may be as high as 60%, accounting for the red mucous membrane color often noted at birth [17]. By 3 days of age, red blood cell counts have decreased dramatically and continue to decrease for approximately 3 weeks [15]. Adult levels for red blood cell count, hemoglobin, and hematocrit are generally not detected in most dogs until 6 months of age, with increases from the 3-week nadir detectable at approximately 2 months of age [15,16]. A similar maturation pattern is noted in the cat [18]. Reference guidelines for the hematologic values of canine and feline neonates may be found in Tables 1 and 2.

Neonatal isoerythrolysis is uncommon in the cat and rare in the dog [16]. In the cat, the phenomenon occurs in association with a type A kitten born to a type B queen that has anti-A alloantibodies (agglutinating and hemolytic) [16]. There is a geographic distribution to type B alloantigen, with the highest prevalence being in Exotic, British short-haired, and Cornish and Devon Rex cats. Despite naturally occurring anti-B alloantibodies in type A queens, isoerythrolysis is not typically noted, most likely because of weak agglutinins and hemolytic activity.

White blood cell parameters in canine and feline neonates are typically consistent with those of their adult counterparts, with feline white blood cell counts being at the low end of the adult reference range at days 7 through 14 [16,18]. One evaluation of Beagle puppies detected a white blood cell count outside the adult reference range during the first 3 days of life; however, whether this is a specific breed- or colony-related phenomenon is unknown [17]. Lymphocytosis may also be noted in the normal neonate [19].

Clinical Implications

During the neonatal period, polychromasia and elevated reticulocyte counts may be noted as fetal red blood cells are replaced [16]. Care must be taken to ensure adequate ectoparasite control, because iron demands are high. Blood loss anemia exacerbates any negative iron balance and may be difficult to distinguish clinically from physiologic anemia; however, the presence of microcytosis is suggestive of iron deficiency anemia. After consideration of the age

Table 1
Hematologic reference values to growing healthy Beagles

Hematologic parameter	Age (in weeks)										
	Birth	1[a]	2[a]	3[a]	4[a]	6[a]	8[a]	12[b]	16[b]	20[b]	24[b]
RBC ($\times 10^6$/µL)	4.7–5.6 (5.1)	3.6–5.9 (4.6)	3.4–4.4 (3.9)	3.5–4.3 (3.8)	3.6–4.9 (4.1)	4.3–5.1 (4.7)	4.5–5.9 (4.9)	6.34	6.38	6.93	7.41
Hemoglobin (g/dL)	14.0–17.0 (15.2)	10.4–17.5 (12.9)	9.0–11.0 (10.0)	8.6–11.6 (9.7)	8.5–10.3 (9.5)	8.5–11.3 (11.2)	10.3–12.5 (11.2)	14.3	15.0	16.0	16.7
PCV %	45.0–52.5 (47.5)	33.0–52.0 (40.5)	29.0–34.0 (31.8)	27.0–37.0 (31.7)	27.0–33.5 (29.9)	26.5–35.5 (32.5)	31.0–39.0 (34.8)	40.9	43.0	44.9	47.6
MCV (fl)	93.0	89.0	81.5	83.0	73.0	69.0	72.0	64.6	67.4	64.8	64.2
MCH (pg)	30.0	28.0	25.5	25.0	23.0	22.0	22.5	22.8	23.5	23.0	22.5
MCHC (%)	32.0	32.0	31.5	31.0	32.0	31.5	32.0	35.3	34.8	35.6	35.1
N-RBC/100 WBC	0–13 (2.3)	0–11 (4.0)	0–6 (2.0)	0–9 (1.6)	0–4 (1.2)	0–0 —	0–1 (0.2)				
Reticulocytes (%)	4.5–9.2 (6.5)	3.8–15.2 (6.9)	4.0–8.4 (6.7)	5.0–9.0 (6.9)	4.6–6.6 (5.8)	2.6–6.2 (4.5)	1.0–6.0 (3.6)				
Total WBC ($\times 10^3$/µL)	6.8–18.4 (12.0)	9.0–23.0 (14.1)	8.1–15.1 (11.7)	6.7–15.1 (11.2)	8.5–16.4 (12.9)	12.6–26.7 (16.3)	12.7–17.3 (15.0)	17.1	16.3	14.6	15.6
Band neutrophils	0–1.5 (0.23)	0–4.8 (0.50)	0–1.2 (0.21)	0–0.5 (0.09)	0–0.3 (0.06)	0–0.3 (0.05)	0–0.3 (0.08)	0.08	0.09	0.02	0.02
Segmented neutrophils	4.4–15.8 (8.6)	3.8–15.2 (7.4)	3.2–10.4 (5.2)	1.4–9.4 (5.1)	3.7–12.8 (7.2)	4.2–17.6 (9.0)	6.2–11.8 (8.5)	9.8	9.0	8.9	9.1
Lymphocytes	0.5–4.2 (1.9)	1.3–9.4 (4.3)	1.5–7.4 (3.8)	2.1–10.1 (5.0)	1.0–8.4 (4.5)	2.8–16.6 (5.7)	3.1–6.9 (5.0)	5.7	5.9	4.5	5.3
Monocytes	0.2–2.2 (0.9)	0.3–2.5 (1.1)	0.2–1.4 (0.7)	0.1–1.4 (0.7)	0.3–1.5 (0.8)	0.5–2.7 (1.1)	0.4–1.7 (1.0)	0.9	0.9	0.8	0.7
Eosinophils	0–1.3 (0.4)	0.2–2.8 (0.8)	0.08–1.8 (0.6)	0.07–0.9 (0.3)	0–0.7 (0.25)	0.1–1.9 (0.5)	0–1.2 (0.4)	0.4	0.4	0.3	0.5
Basophils	0–0.2 (0.01)	0–0.2 (0.01)	0.0	0.0	0–0.15	0.0	0.0				

Abbreviations: MCH, mean corpuscular hemoglobin expressed in picograms; MCHC, mean corpuscular hemoglobin concentration expressed as percentage; MCV, mean corpuscular volume expressed in femtoliters; N-RBC/100 WBC, number of nucleated red blood cells per 100 white blood cells; PCV, packed cell volume; RBC, red blood cells; total WBC, total number of white blood cells.

[a]Normal ranges and/or mean values from Anderson AC, Gee W. Normal blood values in the beagle. Vet Med 1958;53:135.

[b]Mean values from Earl FL, Melvegar BA, Wilson RL. The hemogram and bone marrow profile of norma neonatal and weanling beagle dogs. Lab Anim Sci 1973;23:630.

From Clinkenbeard KD, Cowell RL, Meinkoth JH, et al. The hematopoietic and lymphoid systems. In: Hoskins JD, editor. Veterinary pediatrics: dogs and cats from birth to six months. 3rd edition. Philadelphia: WB Saunders; 2001. p. 301; Table 15-1; with permission.

Table 2
Hematologic reference values for growing healthy cats

Hematologic parameter	Age (in weeks)								
	0–2[a]	2–4[a]	4–6[a]	6–8[a]	8–9[a]	12–13[a]	16–17[a]	20[b]	30[b]
RBC ($\times 10^6$/µL)	5.29 ± 0.24	4.67 ± 0.10	5.89 ± 0.23	6.57 ± 0.26	6.95 ± 0.09	7.43 ± 0.23	8.14 ± 0.27	7.4 ± 0.7	8.0 ± 0.5
Hemoglobin (g/dL)	12.1 ± 0.6	8.7 ± 0.2	8.6 ± 0.3	9.1 ± 0.3	9.8 ± 0.2	10.1 ± 0.3	11.0 ± 0.4	10.7 ± 1.2	12.1 ± 1.8
PCV (%)	35.3 ± 1.7	26.5 ± 0.8	27.1 ± 0.8	29.8 ± 1.3	33.3 ± 0.7	33.1 ± 1.6	34.9 ± 1.1	33.4 ± 3.3	37.1 ± 3.4
MCV (fl)	67.4 ± 1.9	53.9 ± 1.2	45.6 ± 1.3	45.6 ± 1.0	47.8 ± 0.9	44.5 ± 1.8	43.1 ± 1.5	45.0 ± 5.2	46.0 ± 3.5
MCH (pg)	23.0 ± 0.6	18.8 ± 0.8	14.8 ± 0.6	13.9 ± 0.3	14.1 ± 0.2	13.7 ± 0.4	13.5 ± 0.4		
MCHC (%)	34.5 ± 0.8	33.0 ± 0.5	31.9 ± 0.6	30.9 ± 0.5	29.5 ± 0.4	31.3 ± 0.9	31.6 ± 0.8	32.0 ± 2.0	33.0 ± 3.3
Total WBC ($\times 10^3$/µL)	9.67 ± 0.57	15.31 ± 1.21	17.45 ± 1.37	18.07 ± 1.94	23.68 ± 1.89	23.20 ± 3.36	19.70 ± 1.12	15.9 ± 6.0	21.9 ± 6.7
Band neutrophils	0.06 ± 0.02	0.11 ± 0.04	0.20 ± 0.06	0.22 ± 0.08	0.12 ± 0.09	0.15 ± 0.07	0.16 ± 0.07		
Segmented neutrophils	5.96 ± 0.68	6.92 ± 0.77	9.57 ± 0.77	6.75 ± 1.03	11.0 ± 1.41	11.00 ± 1.77	9.74 ± 0.92	9.5 ± 1.27	15.5 ± 1.66
Lymphocytes	3.73 ± 0.52	6.56 ± 0.59	6.41 ± 0.77	9.59 ± 1.57	10.17 ± 1.71	10.46 ± 2.61	8.7 ± 1.06	6.2 ± 1.27	5.7 ± 1.5
Monocytes	0.01 ± 0.01	0.02 ± 0.02	0	0.01 ± 0.01	0.11 ± 0.06	0	0.02 ± 0.02		
Eosinophils	0.96 ± 0.43	1.41 ± 0.16	1.47 ± 0.25	1.08 ± 0.20	2.28 ± 0.31	1.55 ± 0.35	1.00 ± 0.19		
Basophils	0.02 ± 0.01	0	0	0.02 ± 0.02	0	0.03 ± 0.03	0		

Abbreviations: MCH, mean corpuscular hemoglobin expressed in picograms; MCHC, mean corpuscular hemoglobin concentration expressed as percentage; MCV, mean corpuscular volume expressed in femtoliters; PCV, packed cell volume; RBC, red blood cells; total WBC, total number of white blood cells.

[a] Normal ranges *from* Meyers-Wallen VM, Haskins E, Patterson DF. Hematologic values in healthy neonatal, weanling, and juvenile kittens. Am J Vet Res 1984;45:1322.

[b] Normal ranges *from* Anderson L, Wilson R, Hay D. Haematological values in normal cats from four weeks to one year of age. Res Vet Sci 1971;12:579.

From Clikenbeard KD, Cowell RL, Meinkoth JH, et al. The hematopoietic and lymphoid systems. In: Hoskins JD, editor. Veterinary pediatrics: dogs and cats from birth to six months. 3rd edition. Philadelphia: WB Saunders; 2001. p. 302; Table 15-2; with permission.

effect on hematologic parameters, a similar diagnostic approach as used for the adult animal should be applied to the evaluation of red and white blood cell parameters in the neonate. Extramedullary hematopoiesis is commonly noted in the neonate liver [20].

Because of the potential for neonatal isoerythrolysis in the kitten and, rarely, the puppy, any neonate exhibiting acute signs of lethargy, icterus, or hemoglobinuria should be evaluated and aggressively treated. Prevention is based on sire and dam blood typing. The prognosis is poor.

URINARY SYSTEM

There is marked variation in the degree of renal maturation at birth between species [21]. In the dog, the neonatal kidney is morphologically and functionally immature; nephrogenesis continues for at least 2 weeks after birth [22]. There is a paucity of information regarding nephrogenesis in the cat; because of differences noted between other species of the same order (eg, rat, mouse), it would be unwise make any assumption regarding feline neonate renal structure and function from information available regarding the dog.

The canine neonatal kidney is functionally characterized by a low glomerular filtration rate (GFR), renal plasma flow (RPF), filtration fraction (FF), altered para-aminohippurate (PAH) handling, depressed reabsorption of amino acids and phosphate, exaggerated proximal tubule natriuresis, and low concentrating ability [22–26]. Serum creatinine levels and blood urea nitrogen (BUN) concentrations are lower than in the adult animal: typically 0.4 mg/dL and 8 to 10 mg/dL, respectively [19]. Serum phosphorous concentrations are elevated: typically 9 mg/dL because of skeletal growth [19].

Functional alterations in neonatal GFR and RPF occur in parallel but not necessarily in association with the phases of structural development. At birth, arterial pressure is low (50–60 mm Hg); during renal maturation, increased blood pressure and decreased vascular resistance result in an increase in GFR and RPF [22,27]. In the adult dog, the renin-angiotensin system is an important renal autoregulatory mediator; however, in the neonate, renal blood flow is directly correlated with arterial pressure and does not seem to be altered by inhibition of angiotensin until approximately 6 weeks of age [28,29].

Although the ability of the euvolemic canine neonate to excrete sodium is the same as that of an adult dog in a volume-expanded state, despite an absolute increase in sodium excretion, neonatal fractional sodium excretion is decreased in puppies to 3 weeks of age as compared with the adult dog (5% versus 30% in the adult dog) [27,30].

Structurally, unlike the cortical glomerular tufts in the adult dog, the canine neonate kidney has large irregular vessels, with greatest density in the subcapsular zone [22,23]. The cortical peritubular capillary network is immature, with an incomplete subendothelial basement membrane and few fenestrae [31].

With respect to the proximal tubule, there exists a centrifugal distribution of nephron maturation; the oldest and more mature nephrons may be found in the juxtaglomerular zone, whereas nephrons are continually formed for at least the first 2 weeks of life in the subcapsular region [24]. A fourfold increase in outer cortical juxtaglomerular nephrons has been reported during the 4-week neonatal period, with the most rapid increase during the first 8 days of life [32]. Interestingly, it has been speculated that preferential juxtaglomerular blood flow and cortical nephrogenesis result in the canine neonate's relative resistance to the nephrotoxic effects of gentamicin [33]. The canine neonatal proximal tubule is short and composed of smooth cuboidal cells, lacking many of the lateral processes and intracellular organelles noted in the adult [32]. Overall, the canine neonatal proximal tubule lacks the morphologic organization and segmentation of the adult dog, with a reduced surface area and cellular interdigitation [32].

Clinical Implications

Although urine is easy to obtain from the neonate with genital stimulation, the immature nature of the kidney alters interpretation of urinalysis [4]. Low urine specific gravity (1.006–1.0017) is normal, as is the detection of protein, glucose, and various amino acids because of the immaturity of the proximal tubule [34,35]. By 3 weeks of age, urine protein and glucose concentrations approach those of the adult dog, and urine concentration is expected to compare with that of the adult dog by 6 to 8 weeks of age [35,36].

Because the neonatal kidney is less able to concentrate or dilute urine, renal blood flow parallels blood pressure and there is altered sodium excretion by the proximal tubule; fluid therapy should be administered with care to ensure adequate volume maintenance without overhydration or oncotic loading. Recommended daily fluid rates for the canine neonate range from 60 to 180 mL/kg/d [37].

It is interesting to note that in the neonatal rabbit, decreases in body temperature as little as 2°C are able to induce renal vasoconstriction and decrease the GFR [38]. It is possible that a similar phenomenon may occur in canine and feline neonates.

Caution must be exercised when administering renally excreted or metabolized antimicrobials (penicillin, ampicillin, cephalosporins, fluoroquinolones, and aminoglycosides) to neonates [39]. Generally, β-lactam antibiotics are the antimicrobial drug of choice; although the half-life may be prolonged, there is a large therapeutic margin [39]. The authors' preferred antimicrobial in the neonate is ceftiofur, 2.5 mg/kg, subcutaneously every 12 hours for a maximum of 5 days. Because of the altered metabolism of nonsteroidal anti-inflammatory drugs (NSAIDs), the potential for renal toxicity in the neonate is far greater than in the adult animal (see below). Generally, their use is not advised in the neonate.

HEPATOBILIARY SYSTEM

During pregnancy, the maternal placenta supports many functions performed by the liver and biliary system in the adult animal; the ductus venosus shunts blood from the neonatal sinusoid [40]. The canine neonatal liver and biliary system is well described and, similar to that of many species, functionally immature at birth. Descriptions of the feline neonatal hepatobiliary system are lacking.

Canine neonatal bile secretion and control were evaluated in puppies between 0 and 42 days of age and compared with those of adult dogs [40]. Results indicated a significant reduction in bile flow in the newborn puppy as compared with the adult dog and a complete failure of secretin and glucagon to stimulate bile flow at 3 days of age. At 28 days of age, the choleretic effects of secretin and glucagon were 30% to 45% those of the adult dog [40].

In addition to bile flow dynamics, canine neonatal bile contains greater chloride and bicarbonate and less sodium and bile acids as compared with those of the adult dog, whereas serum electrolyte concentrations are similar to those of the adult dog [40]. Bile electrolyte and acid concentrations alter during the neonatal period to approach those of the adult after 8 weeks of age [40].

Despite a relative functional cholestasis in the neonate, serum bile acids may be used to detect hepatocirculatory abnormalities in puppies and kittens as young as 4 weeks of age [41,42]. Alkaline phosphatase (ALP) and gamma-glutamyltransferase (GGT) liver enzyme activities are markedly elevated in the 0- to 2-week-old neonate and moderately elevated after 2 weeks of age [43]. Elevations in ALP and GGT enzyme activity have been attributed to placental, colostral, and intestinal activity [44]. Aspartate aminotransferase (AST) and alanine aminotransferase (ALT) are typically comparable to those of the adult [43]. ALP can be normally elevated during skeletal growth [19].

Postnatal alterations in hepatic microsomal enzyme activities have been evaluated in the canine neonate from 0 to 42 days of age [45,46]. At 4 weeks of age, P_{450}-specific activity was 85% of that seen in an adult dog, whereas adult dog levels of microsomal enzyme activity were not noted until 4.5 months of age [45,46].

Clinical Implications

At birth, the neonate experiences functional cholestasis with altered liver enzyme serum biochemical profiles. Table 3 depicts normal values for hepatic function testing in canine and feline neonates.

Because of the absence of fully developed microsomal and P_{450} enzyme activity in the neonate until 4 to 5 months of age, caution must be exercised when prescribing a medication that requires hepatic metabolism or excretion. Phase I and phase II reactions are reduced in the neonate [39]. Clinically, this results in decreased hepatic metabolism of many drugs, including anticonvulsants (eg, phenobarbital, diazepam) and NSAIDs [39]. The risk of renal injury attributable to NSAID administration in the neonate is greatly increased. Ideally, these medications should be avoided whenever possible because of the paucity of information regarding altered pharmacokinetics in canine and feline neonates. Because a source of serum GGT and ALP is colostrum, detection of serum increases in GGT and ALP in the newborn may be indicative of colostrum intake and potentially passive transfer [44].

Table 3
Normal hepatobiliary biochemical values for canine and feline neonates

Test	Puppies					Kittens		
	1–3 days (n = 30)	2 weeks (n = 14)	4 weeks (n = 7)	8 weeks (n = 8)	Normal adult range	2 weeks (n = 24)	4 weeks (n = 8)	Normal adult range
BSP % 30 min	<5	<5	<5	<5	0–5	ND	ND	0–3
Bile acids (μM/L)	<15	<15	<15	<15	0–15	ND	<10	0–10
Total bilirubin (mg/dL)	0.5 (0.2–1.0)	0.3 (0.1–0.5)	0 (0–0.1)	0.1 (0.1–0.2)	0–0.4	0.3 (0.1–1.0)	0.2 (0.1–0.2)	0–0.2
ALT (IU/L)	69 (17–337)	15 (10–21)	21 (20–22)	21 (9–24)	12–94	18 (11–24)	16 (14–26)	28–91
AST (IU/L)	108 (45–194)	20 (10–40)	18 (14–23)	22 (10–32)	13–56	18 (8–48)	17 (12–24)	9–42
ALP (IU/L)	3845 (618–8760)	236 (176–541)	144 (135–201)	158 (144–177)	4–107	123 (68–269)	111 (90–135)	10–77
GGTP (IU/L)	1111 (163–3558)	24 (4–77)	3 (2–7)	1 (0–7)	0–7	1 (0–3)	2 (0–3)	(0–4)
Total protein (g/dL)	4.1 (3.4–5.2)	3.9 (3.6–4.4)	4.1 (3.9–4.2)	4.6 (3.9–4.8)	5.4–7.4	4.4 (4.0–5.2)	4.8 (4.6–5.2)	5.8–8.0
Albumin (g/dL)	2.1 (1.5–2.8)	1.8 (1.7–2.0)	1.8 (1.0–2.0)	2.5 (2.1–2.7)	2.1–2.3	2.1 (2.0–2.4)	2.3 (2.2–2.4)	2.3–3.0
Cholesterol (mg/dL)	136 (112–204)	282 (223–344)	328 (266–352)	155 (111–258)	103–299	229 (164–443)	361 (222–434)	150–270
Glucose (mg/dL)	88 (52–127)	129 (111–146)	109 (86–115)	145 (134–272)	65–110	117 (76–129)	110 (99–112)	63–144

Abbreviations: ALP, alkaline phosphatase; ALT alanine aminotransferase; AST, aspartate aminotransferase; BSP, sulfobromophthalein; GGTP, gamma-glutamyltranspeptidase; ND, not determined.

Data from Center SA, Hornbuckle WE, New York State College of Veterinary Medicine, Cornell University, 1987; reprinted from Center SA, Hornbuckle WE, Hoskins JD. The liver and pancreas. In: Hoskins JD, editor. Veterinary pediatrics—dogs and cats from birth to six months. 2nd edition. Philadelphia: WB Saunders; 1995. p. 189–225.

From Johnston SD, Root Kustritz MV, Olson PNS. The neonate—from birth to weaning. In: Canine and feline theriogenology. 1st edition. Philadelphia: WB Saunders; 2001. p. 151; Table 8-3; with permission.

GASTROINTESTINAL SYSTEM

Dentition eruption in the neonate first occurs at 2 to 3 weeks of age; all dentitious teeth should be present by 12 weeks of age (Table 4) [19]. At birth, the gastrointestinal tract is sterile and characterized by a neutral gastric pH and a time-dependent increased permeability of the intestinal mucosa, which decreases dramatically after 10 hours [47,48]. Normal nursing pup feces are semiformed and tan in color [19].

In one study evaluating the intestinal motility of the canine neonate small bowel, it was noted that electrical activity commenced at day 40, suggesting that motility before this time is dependent on pressure gradients rather than on intestinal motility [49]. Body temperature is known to have a dramatic effect on gastrointestinal movement in the neonate; at rectal temperatures less than 94°F, ileus develops, decreasing the willingness to nurse and predisposing tube-fed puppies to aspiration and subsequent pneumonia [19].

Clinical Implications

Care should be taken to ensure adequate environmental conditions to maintain normal body temperature in neonates so as to minimize gastrointestinal ileus. Because of increased gastrointestinal permeability and neutral gastric pH in the immediate postnatal period, care must be taken if administering oral drug therapy because of altered absorption [39].

IMMUNE SYSTEM

Neonatal mortality during the first 3 weeks of age is reported to range between 7% and 34%, with septicemia a major cause of death [37,50]. Although the bitch and queen demonstrate endotheliochorial placentation, there are differences between the species with respect to transplacental antibody transfer. In the cat, as much as 25% of a kitten's serum antibodies may be derived via transplacental antibody transfer [51]. In comparison, 5% to 10% of canine neonatal

Table 4	
Normal tooth eruption times for the puppy	
Age	**Deciduous teeth[a,b]**
3–4 weeks	Canine (C)
4–5 weeks	Incisor (I) 1, incisor 2, premolar (P) 2, premolar 3
5–6 weeks	Incisor 3, premolar 4
	Permanent teeth[c]
4–5 months	Incisor 1, incisor 2, incisor 3, premolar 1, molar (M)1
5–6 months	Canine, premolar 2, premolar 3, premolar 4, molar 2
6–7 months	Molar 3

[a]Some adult dogs may lack first and second premolars; last molars may be absent in brachycephalic breeds.
[b]Dental formula for deciduous teeth: 2(I 3/3; C 1/1; P 3/3) = 28.
[c]Dental formula for permanent teeth: 2(I 3/3; C 1/1; P 4/4; M 2/3) = 42.
From Johnston SD, Root Kustritz MV, Olson PNS. The neonate—from birth to weaning. In: Canine and feline theriogenology. 1st edition. Philadelphia: WB Saunders; 2001. p. 153; Table 8-6; with permission.

serum antibodies are derived from transplacental transfer [52]. At birth, canine and feline neonates are antibody deficient and immunologically incompetent, with the acquisition of passive immunity requiring adequate ingestion and absorption of colostrum during the first 24 hours of life; absorption of antibodies decreases markedly after 12 hours [19,53].

In the dog, the highest concentration of immunoglobulin isotype in colostrum is IgG, followed by IgA and IgM. The total immunoglobulin concentration decreases dramatically from 15 mg/mL at parturition to 3 mg/mL on the following 2 days as milk replaces colostrum in the mammary gland [54,55]. In an evaluation of five newborn puppies, serum IgG serum concentrations were noted to increase from 35 to 3366 mg/dL, IgM from 8 to 71 mg/dL, and IgA from 0 to 575 mg/dL after colostrum administration [56]. Nasal immunoglobulin isotypes in the dog were recently characterized, with IgG being the predominant isotype during the first 3 days of life and after 4 weeks and an altering IgG/IgA ratio between weeks 1 and 3 because of decreasing IgG concentrations [57]. IgM was only detectable in a small portion of neonatal dogs during the first week of life [57].

Provided adequate ingestion of quality colostrum, the puppy and kitten are protected by maternally derived immunoglobulins during the neonatal period [19]. Antigenic stimulation of 1-day-old puppies has shown that puppies are capable of producing challenge-specific antibodies within 2 weeks and, with repeated challenge at 40 days, a secondary immune response; however, T-cell mitogenesis and differentiation and phagocytic cell function systems may not be fully mature [19,58].

Clinical Implications

When colostral intake is not possible or is of questionable quality, pooled adult dog serum (22 mL/kg administered subcutaneously) may be administered to elevate serum immunoglobulin concentrations in the puppy [56,59]. In the kitten, 15 mL per kitten (approximately 150 mL/kg) administered subcutaneously or intraperitoneally has been shown to correct IgG deficiency successfully in colostrum-deprived kittens [60].

METABOLISM

The normal birth weight of a kitten is 100 ± 10 g; that of a puppy is breed dependent, generally 500 ± 150 g for a medium-sized dog. Birth weights lower than 90 g in the kitten or 300 g in the medium-sized dog are associated with an increased risk of neonatal mortality, which is most likely associated with negative effects of chilling (higher body surface area/mass ratio) and the ability to nurse and maintain glucose concentrations [61,62]. Generally, there is a similar pattern of growth among different breeds of dogs, with the most rapid weight gain occurring during the first 12 weeks of life [4]. Puppies and kittens should gain, on average, 10% of their body weight each day for the first few weeks of life.

Unlike their homeothermic adult counterparts, neonates are poikilothermic; however, they have well developed behavioral heat-seeking responses that enable them to maintain a stable rectal temperature provided that sources of heat are available [62]. The importance of this phenomenon is highlighted by evaluation of puppy responses to environmental temperature; hypothermia induced by cooling environment exposure disappears within 1 hour provided that one of the following is provided: the dam, a box containing a hot water bottle at 110°F, or an incubator at 85°F [63]. Shivering and vasoconstrictive reflexes are not functional in the newborn [19]. Physiologic responses noted during hypothermia include bradycardia, cardiovascular failure, neuronal injury, and ileus [19]. According to Crighton [62,63], a healthy newborn puppy can survive up to 12 hours of hypothermia with adequate warming and return to the dam.

Normal rectal temperatures in the puppy are 95°F to 99°F (week 1) and 97°F to 100°F (weeks 2 and 3); at weaning, rectal temperature approaches that of the adult [19]. Similar temperatures are noted for the kitten [64]. Recommended environmental temperatures for the puppy and kitten may be found in Table 5.

At birth, the neonate must transition from placental support to endogenous food stores for glucose production. During the first 3 to 24 hours, hepatic glycogen stores decline by more than 50% and there is a shift from glycogenolysis to a mixture of glycogenolysis and gluconeogenesis [65,66]. For maintenance of blood glucose concentrations, regular feeding is required to provide an energy source. In addition to regular nursing, the dam's nutritional state must be adequate; puppies of starved dams experience a temporary 24-hour decrease in glucose production rate, after which adaptation occurs [65].

Clinical Implications

Neonates are susceptible to a wide variety of toxic, environmental, infectious, and congenital insults; however, the ability for them to respond is limited. One of the first signs of illness in kittens and puppies is a failure to gain weight; this often noted well before any other clinical signs of disease are present. Twice-daily weighing of neonates during the first week(s) of life dramatically increases the early detection of illness, ensures adequate intervention in a timely manner so as to prevent poor weight gain, and has a positive impact on neonatal mortality.

Table 5
Environmental temperature guidelines for canine and feline neonates

Age (days)	Temperature (°F)
0–7	85–90
8–14	80
15–28	80
29–35	70–75
35	70

Data from Monson WJ. Orphan rearing of puppies and kittens. Vet Clin North Am Small Anim Pract 1987;17:567–76; and Johnston SD, Root Kustritz MV, Olson PNS. The neonate—from birth to weaning. In: Canine and feline theriogenology. 1st edition. Philadelphia: WB Saunders; 2001. p. 147; Table 8-1.

Environmental conditions should be maintained to ensure adequate thermo-regulation without excessive heat; if humidity levels are high, the ambient temperature should be adjusted. The recommended humidity level is 55% to 65% [64].

Attention should be paid to dam nutrition and frequency of neonate nursing to ensure that neonates are receiving adequate energy sources to maintain serum glucose concentrations.

OCULAR SYSTEM

The eyelids typically separate between 5 and 14 days of age in feline and canine neonates. The cornea appears slightly cloudy for the first 2 to 4 weeks of life because of increased water content, and the iris is typically bluish gray because of low pigmentation [67]. Hyaloid artery remnants may be visible attached to the posterior lens at the time of eyelid separation [67].

Retinal vascular development is incomplete at birth in the dog and cat, with the puppy retina being more completely vascularized than the kitten retina (60% versus 12%). Both species exhibit peripheral retinal vascularization by 14 days of age [68,69].

Clinical Implications

Evaluation of the neonatal eye is limited until such a time as the eyelids separate. Pupillary light reflexes are dependent on retinal development, which typically occurs around 2 weeks of age. Funduscopy reveals a blue-gray tapetum until 4 to 7 months of age [67].

NEUROLOGIC SYSTEM

For a detailed discussion regarding the development and evaluation of the nervous system in the neonate, the reader is referred to the article by Lavely in this issue.

References

[1] Adelman RD, Wright J. Systolic blood pressure and heart rate in the growing beagle puppy. Dev Pharmacol Ther 1985;8:396–401.

[2] Magrini F. Haemodynamic determinants of the arterial blood pressure rise during growth in conscious puppies. Cardiovasc Res 1978;12:422–8.

[3] Mace SE, Levy MN. Neural control of heart rate: a comparison between puppies and adult animals. Pediatr Res 1983;17:491–5.

[4] Fox MW. Developmental physiology and behavior. In: Fox MW, Himwich WA, editors. Canine pediatrics. Springfield (MO): Charles C Thomas; 1966. p. 22–5.

[5] Swann HG, Christian JJ, Hamilton C. The process of anoxic death in newborn pups. Surg Gynecol Obstet 1954;99:5–8.

[6] Finley JP, Kelly C. Heart rate and respiratory patterns in mild hypoxia in unanaesthetized newborn mammals. Can J Physiol Pharmacol 1985;64:122–4.

[7] Fox MW. The ontogeny of behavior and neurologic responses in the dog. J Anim Behav 1964;12:301–10.

[8] Haddad GG, Mellins RB. Hypoxia and respiratory control in early life. Ann Rev Physiol 1984;46:629–43.

[9] Haddad GG, Gandhi R, Mellins RB. Maturation of ventilatory response to hypoxia in puppies during sleep. J Appl Physiol 1982;52:309–14.

[10] Blanco CE, Hanson MA, Johnson P, et al. Breathing pattern of kittens during hypoxia. J Appl Physiol 1984;56:12–7.

[11] Fisher JT, Brundage KL, Waldron MA, et al. Vagal cholinergic innervation of the airways in newborn cat and dog. J Appl Physiol 1990;69:1525–31.

[12] Waldron MA, Fisher JT. Differential effects of CO_2 and hypoxia on bronchomotor tone in the newborn dog. Respir Physiol 1988;72:271–82.

[13] Fisher JT, Waldron MA, Armstrong CJ. Effects of hypoxia on lung mechanics in the newborn cat. Can J Physiol Pharmacol 1987;65:1234–8.

[14] Lelli JL, Drongowski RA, Coran AG, et al. Hypoxia-induced bacterial translocation in the puppy. J Pediatr Surg 1992;27:974–82.

[15] Ederstrom HE, DeBoer B. Changes in the blood of the dog with age. Anat Rec 1946;94: 663–70.

[16] Clinkenbeard KD, Cowell RL, Meinkoth JH, et al. The hematopoietic and lymphoid systems. In: Hoskins JD, et al, editors. Veterinary pediatrics: dogs and cats from birth to six months. 3rd edition. Philadelphia: WB Saunders; 2001. p. 301–43.

[17] Shifrine M, Munn SL, Rosenblatt LS, et al. Hematologic changes to 60 days of age in clinically normal beagles. Lab Anim Sci 1973;23:894–8.

[18] Windle WF, Sweet M, Whitehead WH. Some aspects of prenatal and postnatal development of the blood in the cat. Anat Rec 1940;78:321–32.

[19] Johnston SD, Root Kustritz MV, Olson PNS. The neonate—from birth to weaning. In: Canine and feline theriogenology. 1st edition. Philadelphia: WB Saunders; 2001. p. 146–67.

[20] Hoskins JD. The liver and pancreas. In: Hoskins JD, editor. Veterinary pediatrics: dogs and cats from birth to six months. 3rd edition. Philadelphia: WB Saunders; 2001. p. 200–24. [Table 15-1].

[21] Zoetis T, Hurtt ME. Species comparison of anatomical and functional renal development. Birth Defects Res B Dev Reprod Toxicol 2003;68:111–20.

[22] Evan AP, Stoeckel JA, Loemker V, et al. Development of the intrarenal vascular system of the puppy kidney. Anat Rec 1979;194:187–200.

[23] Olbing H, Blaufox MD, Aschinberg LC, et al. Postnatal changes in renal glomerular blood flow distribution in puppies. J Clin Invest 1973;52:2885–95.

[24] Hay DA, Evan AP. Maturation of the proximal tubule in the puppy kidney: a comparison to the adult. Anat Rec 1979;195:273–300.

[25] Kleinman LI, Banks RO. Pressure natriuresis during saline expansion in newborn and adult dogs. Am J Physiol 1984;246:F828–34.

[26] Kleinman LI, Reuter JH. Renal response of the newborn dog to a saline load: the role of intrarenal blood flow and distribution. J Physiol 1974;239:225–36.

[27] Kleinman LI. Developmental renal physiology. Physiologist 1982;25:104–10.

[28] Kleinman LI, Reuter JH. Maturation of glomerular blood flow distribution in the newborn dog. J Physiol 1973;228:91–103.

[29] Jose PA, Slotkoff LM, Montgomery S, et al. Autoregulation of renal blood flow in the puppy. Am J Physiol 1975;229:983–8.

[30] Aladjem M, Spitzer A, Goldsmith DI. The relationship between intravascular volume expansion and natriuresis in developing puppies. Pediatr Res 1982;16:840–5.

[31] Evan AP, Hay DA. Ultrastructure of the developing vascular system in the puppy kidney. Anat Rec 1981;199:481–9.

[32] Tavani N, Calcagno P, Zimmet S, et al. Ontogeny of single nephron filtration distribution in canine puppies. Pediatr Res 1980;14:799–802.

[33] Cowan RH, Jukkola AF, Arant BS, et al. Pathophysiologic evidence of gentamicin nephrotoxicity in neonatal puppies. Pediatr Res 1980;14:1204–11.

[34] Jezyk PF. Screening for inborn errors of metabolism in dogs and cats. In: Hommes FA, editor. Models for the study of inborn errors of metabolism. 1st edition. Amsterdam: Elsevier Science; 1979. p. 11–8.

[35] Bovee KC, Jezyk PF, Segal SC. Postnatal development of renal tubular amino acid reabsorption in canine pups. Am J Vet Res 1984;45:830–2.

[36] Fettman MJ, Aleen TA. Developmental aspects of fluid and electrolyte metabolism and renal function in neonates. Compend Contin Educ Pract Vet 1991;13:392–7.

[37] Mosier JE. Canine pediatrics: the neonate. Proc Am Anim Hosp Assoc 1981;48:339–47.

[38] Toth-Heyn P, Drukker A, Guignard JP. The stressed neonatal kidney: from pathophysiology to clinical management of neonatal vasomotor nephropathy. Pediatr Nephrol 2000;14:227–39.

[39] Boothe DM, Bucheler J. Drug and blood component therapy and neonatal isoerythrolysis. In: Hoskins JD, editor. Veterinary pediatrics: dogs and cats from birth to six months. 3rd edition. Philadelphia: WB Saunders; 2001. p. 35–56.

[40] Tavolini N. Bile secretion and its control in the newborn puppy. Pediatr Res 1986;20: 203–8.

[41] Center SA, Baldwin BH, de Lahunta A, et al. Evaluation of serum bile acid concentrations for the diagnosis of portosystemic anomalies in the dog and cat. J Am Vet Med Assoc 1985;186:1090–4.

[42] Meyer DJ. Liver function tests in dogs with portosystemic shunts: measurement of serum bile acid concentrations. J Am Vet Med Assoc 1986;188:168–9.

[43] Center SA, Hornbuckle WE, Hoskins JD. The liver and pancreas. In: Hoskins JD, editor. Veterinary pediatrics: dogs and cats from birth to six months. 2nd edition. Philadelphia: WB Saunders; 1995. p. 189–225.

[44] Center SA, Randolph JF, ManWarren T, et al. Effect of colostrum ingestion of gamma-glutamylaminotransferase and alkaline phosphatase activity in neonatal pups. Am J Vet Res 1991;52:499–504.

[45] Tavolini N. Postnatal changes in hepatic microsomal enzyme activities in the puppy. Biol Neonate 1985;47:305–16.

[46] Peters EL, Farber TM, Heider A, et al. The development of drug-metabolizing enzymes in the young dog. Fed Proc Am Soc Biol 1971;30:560.

[47] Heinmann G. Enteral absorption and bioavailability in children in relation to age. Eur J Clin Pharmacol 1980;18:43–50.

[48] Gillette DD, Filkins M. Factors affecting antibody transfer in the newborn puppy. Am J Physiol 1966;210:419–22.

[49] Bueno L, Ruckebusch Y. Perinatal development of intestinal myoelectrical activity in dogs and sheep. Am J Physiol 1979;237:E61–7.

[50] Scott FW, Geissinger C. Kitten mortality survey. Feline Pract 1978;8:31–4.

[51] Harding SK, Bruner DW, Bryant IW. The transfer of antibodies from the mother to her newborn kittens. Cornell Vet 1961;51:535–9.

[52] Johnston SD, Root Kustritz MV, Olson PNS. Canine pregnancy. In: Canine and feline theriogenology. 1st edition. Philadelphia: WB Saunders; 2001. p. 66–104.

[53] Gillette DD, Filkins M. Factors affecting antibody transfer in the newborn puppy. Am J Physiol 1966;210:419–22.

[54] Reynolds HY, Johnson JS. Quantification of canine immunoglobulins. J Immunol 1970;105: 698–703.

[55] Heddle RJ, Rowley D. Immunochemical characterization of dog serum, parotid saliva, colostrums, milk and small bowel fluid. Immunology 1975;29:185–95.

[56] Bouchard G, Plata-Madrid H, Youngquist RS, et al. Absorption of an alternate source of immunoglobulin in pups. Am J Vet Res 1992;53:230–3.

[57] Schäfer-Somi S, Bär-Schadler S, Aurich J. Immunoglobulins in nasal secretions of dog puppies from birth to six weeks of age. Res Vet Sci 2005;78:143–50.

[58] Shifrine M, Smith JB, Bulgin MS, et al. Response of canine fetuses and neonates to antigenic stimulation. J Immunol 1971;107:965–70.

[59] Poffenbarger EM, Olson PN, Chandler ML, et al. Use of adult dog serum as a substitute for colostrum in the neonatal dog. Am J Vet Res 1991;52:1221–4.

[60] Levy JK, Crawford PC, Collante WR, et al. Use of adult cat serum to correct failure of passive transfer in kittens. J Am Vet Med Assoc 2001;219:1401–5.
[61] Johnston SD, Root Kustritz MV, Olson PNS. The post partum period in the cat. In: Canine and feline theriogenology. 1st edition. Philadelphia: WB Saunders; 2001. p. 438–52.
[62] Chrighton GW. Thermal regulation in the newborn dog. Mod Vet Pract 1969;(Feb):35–46.
[63] Crighton GW. Thermal balance in new-born puppies. Vet Rec 1962;74:474–81.
[64] Mosier JE. The puppy from birth to six weeks. Vet Clin North Am Small Anim Pract 1978;8: 79–100.
[65] Kliegman RM, Miettinen EL, Adam PAJ. Fetal and neonatal responses to maternal canine starvation: circulating fuels and neonatal glucose production. Pediatr Res 1981;15: 945–51.
[66] Kliegman RM, Morton S. The metabolic response of the canine neonate to twenty-four hours of fasting. Metabolism 1987;36:521–6.
[67] Hoskins JD, Glaze MB. The eye. In: Hoskins JD, editor. Veterinary pediatrics: dogs and cats from birth to six months. 3rd edition. Philadelphia: WB Saunders; 2001. p. 270–99.
[68] Flower RW, McLeod DS, Lutty GA, et al. Postnatal retinal vascular development of the puppy. Invest Ophthalmol Vis Sci 1985;26:957–68.
[69] Flower RW. Perinatal ocular physiology and ROP in the experimental animal model. Doc Ophthalmol 1990;74:153–62.

Vet Clin Small Anim 36 (2006) 461–474

VETERINARY CLINICS
SMALL ANIMAL PRACTICE

Recent Advances in Small Animal Genetics

Danika L. Bannasch, DVM, PhD[a,b,*], Angela M. Hughes, DVM[a]

[a]Veterinary Medical Teaching Hospital, School of Veterinary Medicine, One Shields Avenue,
University of California at Davis, Davis, CA 95616, USA
[b]Department of Population Health and Reproduction, School of Veterinary Medicine,
One Shields Avenue, University of California at Davis, Davis, CA 95616, USA

SEQUENCING THE CANINE GENOME

The unique breed structure of the domestic dog creates a tremendous opportunity to investigate the genes involved in disease susceptibility, morphology, and behavior, because many breeds were created to enhance certain desired traits by mating closely related individuals. A better understanding of the role of genes, particularly in the development of disease, cannot only improve the health of our canine companions but can lead to insights into human health and disease. This is particularly important, because dogs are more closely related to human beings than most domestic species, including mice.

To assist researchers investigating the genetics of canine traits and diseases, an effort was undertaken to sequence the dog genome. To understand better how this was done, let's step back a moment and review the basics of the canine genetic structure.

The basic blueprint for life in most organisms, the genetic material, is DNA. DNA is comprised of two polymer strands of bases: A, T, G, and C. These bases align to form complementary base pairings such that A always pairs with T and G always pairs with C (Fig. 1). These strands can be completely separated and replicated in preparation for cellular division. Alternatively, these strands can be partially separated, transcribed into RNA, and translated into functional proteins. The DNA sequence of the canine genome is broken up into 38 autosomes and a pair of sex chromosomes, X and Y. Each chromosome contains a variety of genes as well as "filler" DNA that does not encode for proteins but may be involved in the degree to which each gene is expressed.

Although a handful of disease- or trait-causing mutations have been identified by examining obvious candidate genes (genes that cause a similar

*Corresponding author. Department of Population Health and Reproduction, School of Veterinary Medicine, One Shields Avenue, University of California at Davis, Davis, CA 95616, USA. E-mail address: dlbannasch@ucdavis.edu (D.L. Bannasch).

0195-5616/06/$ – see front matter
doi:10.1016/j.cvsm.2005.12.004

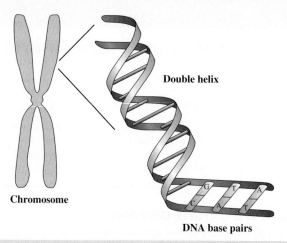

Fig. 1. DNA, the genetic blueprint, is contained in chromosomes. Each chromosome consists of two polymer strands of complimentary paired DNA bases (A, T, G, and C) in the form of a double helix.

phenotype in another species, such as human beings or mice), including X-linked severe combined immunodeficiency and pyruvate kinase deficiency, there are many other genetic diseases, such as hip dysplasia, cancer, and many immune-mediated diseases, that do not have an explicit candidate gene or involve multiple genes [1,2]. Additionally, researchers interested in a particular gene often had to determine the DNA sequence of that particular gene, which can be a rather tedious and time-consuming process. Thus, to assist and speed up the hunt to find the genes that cause these diseases and traits of interest, it was proposed that the dog's genome be sequenced [3].

With funding from the National Institutes of Health (NIH), the sequencing of a female Boxer named Tasha was principally conducted at the Broad Institute, formerly the Whitehead Institute/Massachusetts Institute of Technology (MIT) Center for Genome Research. Tasha was specifically chosen as the "model" dog because she was the least heterozygous, meaning that each pair of chromosomes was more likely to be identical at each base than those of any of the numerous other dogs considered. As a result, it is easier for the scientists to determine the appropriate base at each location in the sequence. For the actual sequencing, they used a whole-genome shotgun (WGS) approach, which, simply put, cuts the entire genome into smaller and more manageable pieces; determines the sequence of each piece; and using overlap between the pieces, then realigns the entire sequence (Fig. 2). The original compiled dog genome sequence was released to the public in July 2004, and, to date, approximately 98% of the dog genome has been sequenced.

Although most of the actual sequence for the dog genome is now known, we are still far from understanding what it all means. Researchers are in the process of meticulously examining the genomic sequence and trying to determine

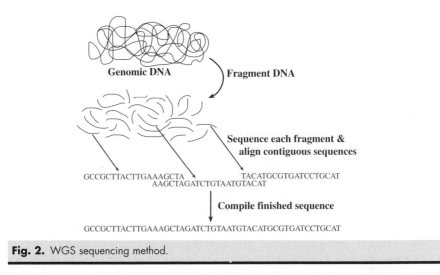

Fig. 2. WGS sequencing method.

which portions encode for genes and which are important for controlling gene expression. The information obtained about the canine genome not only greatly improves our ability to examine the genetic basis for traits and diseases by providing a basic blueprint to work with; it also allows scientists studying the structure of the genome and the evolution of species to compare the dog genome with that of other mammals, including human beings.

The implications for veterinary medicine of sequencing the dog genome are numerous, including increased understanding of disease and trait pathogenesis, improved diagnostic capabilities using genetic testing, and, ultimately, production of healthier companion animals.

SEQUENCING THE FELINE GENOME

For many of the same reasons that the canine genome was sequenced, the feline genome is currently being sequenced as well. Again, cats share our environment, receive advanced medical care, and experience unique inherited (eg, polycystic kidney disease) and infectious (eg, feline leukemia virus [FeLV], feline immunodeficiency virus [FIV]) diseases, which make them an excellent model species, particularly for human diseases [4].

As opposed to dogs, where selective breeding for many centuries has created hundreds of distinct breeds, most cat breeds have been created within the past century and were often based on single gene traits, such as coat color or type. Thus, cat breeds and, consequently, their genes tend to be much more homogeneous than dog breeds, resulting in fewer breed-specific genetic diseases and morphologic differences.

The cat genome is contained in 18 pairs of chromosomes plus the sex chromosomes. This genomic sequence will be used largely for comparative purposes with other mammalian species; thus, it has been decided that the cat genome is not going to be sequenced quite as extensively as the dog genome.

Nonetheless, it will provide a significant amount of specific sequence and general genomic information. The cat sequencing efforts are currently underway through a collaborative effort between Agencourt Biosciences Corporation and the Broad Institute with funding from the NIH, using the same WGS method described previously.

GENETIC TESTS

Thanks to recent advances in technology and the resources available to the research community, the genetic basis for many diseases and traits has been identified for dogs and cats. Please refer to the chapter titled "Canine Molecular Genetic Testing in the March 2001 issue of *Veterinary Clinics of North America: Small Animal Practice* [5] for a discussion of molecular genetic testing, including sampling, individual identification and parentage analysis, mutation testing, and linked marker testing. There are currently more than 100 breed- and DNA-based testing combinations for inherited diseases and traits in dogs (Table 1), and more than a dozen such combinations are available for cats (Table 2). Although these are comprehensive lists of the commercial tests available at this time, they will certainly continue to grow as new discoveries are made. Veterinarians are urged to contact one of the genetics services available at veterinary schools for the latest information regarding available DNA-based tests.

GENE THERAPY

The rapid advancements in the understanding of the molecular basis of inherited disease in dogs, and to a lesser degree in cats, provide opportunities for correction of those diseases using gene therapy. Gene therapy is a treatment modality that uses the introduction of genes (DNA) or RNA by various means to restore the normal or near-normal phenotype to an individual with an inherited disease. Generally, this therapy would only alter somatic tissue or the organ responsible for the defect. It does not change the animal's ability to pass the disease to its offspring. Although gene therapy may seem particularly futuristic as a treatment option in veterinary medicine, many advances have been made in gene therapy, because dogs and cats serve as animal models for human disease. The US Food and Drug Administration is much more likely to consider allowing gene therapy to proceed to clinical trials in people if the same disease has been corrected in an animal model with minimal side effects. The bonus to veterinary medicine is that once the protocols have been worked out in experimental environments, the treatments could be used for privately owned patients.

The first report of successful gene therapy in dogs occurred in 1993 when sustained partial correction of hemophilia B (factor IX deficiency) was obtained using recombinant retroviral vectors [52]. Since that time, there have been dozens of reports of successful gene therapy for hemophilia B and hemophilia A in dogs using many different types of vector delivery systems [53]. The work in the dog models of hemophilia has paved the way for clinical trials in human beings.

One of the most exciting advances in gene therapy is the ability to restore vision in cases of inherited blindness. In 2001, Acland and colleagues [54] reported on the restoration of vision in dogs with a naturally occurring mutation in the RPE65 gene. These initial experiments were performed in puppies; Narfstrom and coworkers [55] have demonstrated vision restoration in adult dogs using a similar vector delivery system and subretinal injections. Even more promising is the result that injection into one eye was able to restore vision to the contralateral eye as well. Successful gene therapy has also been performed in Collies with gray collie syndrome or cyclic neutropenia. A lentivirus vector was used to provide recombinant granulocyte colony-stimulating factor through intramuscular injections. Neutrophil counts remained elevated for 17 months after injections and the "affected" dog was able to live outside a pathogen-free environment [56]. Gene therapy has also been successful for lysosomal storage diseases in dog and cat models, paving the way for human clinical trials for these severely debilitating diseases [57,58].

Gene therapy can also be used to treat diseases without a defined inherited basis. Recently, Choi and colleagues [59] used a nonviral peptide vector to treat systemic lupus erythematosus in an induced canine model system. This promising research opens up the possibility that gene therapy treatments might be made available for diseases without a defined inherited basis once the pathogenesis of those diseases is well understood.

CLONING

A clone refers to an individual developed from a single somatic (nongerm) cell from a single parent. The clone and the parent have the exact same genetic material. The first domestic cat was cloned by somatic cell nuclear transfer in 2002 [60]. Since that time, a number of different research laboratories have cloned domestic cats as well as African Wildcats using domestic cats as surrogates [61,62]. Recently, a dog was cloned by researchers in South Korea [63]. Dog cloning is a much less efficient process than cat cloning or cloning of other domestic animals. This is partially attributable to the fact that dogs ovulate infrequently and partly attributable to the fact that dogs produce primary oocytes that are immature and are not ready to be fertilized for 2 to 5 days.

Cloned domestic animals have been extremely useful research tools and should continue to have great benefit to research in the future. One of the most interesting questions that can be addressed by clones is the effect that genetics versus environment has on disease phenotypes. Cloning of domestic cats is now being offered on a commercial basis to pet owners (with the recent successful cloning of a dog, we assume that dog cloning will also become commercially available soon). The commercialization of pet cloning brings up important ethical and medical considerations that should be considered by veterinarians.

Veterinarians play an integral part in the cloning process and can provide clients with more information about cloning because they are the ones required to obtain the tissue samples used in the process of cloning. Veterinarians collect the tissue biopsies that are stored by companies until the client wishes to pursue

Table 1
Commercial tests available for inherited diseases and traits in dogs as of August 31, 2005

Disease/trait	Breeds	MOI	Type of test	Test laboratory[a]	References
Canine cyclic neutropenia	Collie (Rough and Smooth), gray	AR	MT	H	[6]
Canine globoid cell leukodystrophy	Cairn Terrier, West Highland White Terrier	AR	MT	H	[7]
Canine leukocyte adhesion deficiency	Irish Setter, Irish Red and White Setter	AR	MT	O, H	[8,9]
Canine muscular dystrophy	Golden Retriever	X-linked	MT	H	[10]
Coat color	Various breeds			V, H	
Cobalamin malabsorption	Australian Shepherd, Giant Schnauzer	AR	MT	M, P	[11]
Collie eye anomaly/choroidal hypoplasia	Australian Shepherd, Border Collie, Collie (Rough and Smooth), Lancashire Heeler, Shetland Sheepdog	?	MT	O	[12,13]
Cone degeneration	German Short-Haired Pointer	AR	MT	O	[14]
Congenital hypothyroidism with goiter	Rat Terrier, Toy Fox Terrier	AR	MT	M, P, H	[15]
Congenital stationary night blindness	Briard	AR	MT	O, H	[16]
Copper toxicosis	Bedlington Terrier	AR	LMT	V	[17,18]
Cystinuria	Labrador Retriever, Newfoundland	AR	MT	P, V, O, H	[19]
Factor VII deficiency	Beagle	AR	MT	P	
Fucosidosis	English Springer Spaniel	AR	MT	P	[20]
GM1 gangliosidosis	Portuguese Water Dog	AR	MT	H	[21]
Glycogen storage disease IIIa	Curly-Coated Retriever	AR	MT	M	[22,23]
Hemophilia B	Airedale Terrier, Bull Terrier, Labrador Retriever, Lhasa Apso	X-linked	MT	H	
Mucopolysaccharidosis IIIB	Schipperke	AR	MT	P	[24]
Mucopolysaccharidosis VI	Miniature Pinscher	AR	MT	P	[25]
Mucopolysaccharidosis VII	German Shepherd Dog	AR	MT	P	[26]
Multidrug (ivermectin) sensitivity	Collie (Rough and Smooth)	?	MT	W	[27,28]
Myotonia congenita	Schnauzer (Miniature)	AR	MT	P, H	[29,30]
Narcolepsy	Dachshund, Doberman Pinscher, Labrador Retriever	AR	MT	O, H	
Neuronal ceroid lipofuscinosis	Border Collie	AR	MT	O	[31]

Disease	Breeds	MOI	Test	Labs	Refs
Phosphofructokinase deficiency	American Cocker Spaniel, English Cocker Spaniel, English Springer Spaniel	AR	MT	P, V, O, H	[32,33]
Progressive retinal atrophy: dominant	Bullmastiff, Mastiff	AD	MT	O	[34]
Progressive retinal atrophy: prcd	American Cocker Spaniel, American Eskimo Dog, Australian Cattle Dog, Australian Stumpy Tail Cattle Dog, Chesapeake Bay Retriever, Chinese Crested, English Cocker Spaniel, Entlebucher Mountain Dog, Labrador Retriever, Nova Scotia Duck Tolling Retriever, Poodle (Miniature and Toy), Portuguese Water Dog	AR	MT	O	
Progressive retinal atrophy: rcd1	Irish Setter, Irish Red and White Setter	AR	MT	V, O, H	[35–37]
Progressive retinal atrophy: rcd1a	Sloughi	AR	MT	O	[38]
Progressive retinal atrophy: rcd3	Cardigan Welsh Corgi	AR	MT	O, H	[39,40]
Progressive retinal atrophy: type A	Schnauzer (Miniature)	?	MT	O	
Progressive retinal atrophy: x-linked	Samoyed, Siberian Husky	X-linked	MT	O	
Pyruvate kinase deficiency	Basenji, Beagle, Cairn Terrier, Chihuahua, Dachshund, American Eskimo Dog, West Highland White Terrier	AR	MT	P, V, O, H	[2,41–43]
Renal dysplasia	Lhasa Apso, Shih Tzu, Soft-Coated Wheaten Terrier	?	LMT	V	
Severe combined immunodeficiency	Basset Hound, Cardigan Welsh Corgi	X-linked	MT	P	[1,44]
von Willebrand's disease type 1	Bernese Mountain Dog, Doberman Pinscher, Drentsche Patrijshond, German Pinscher, Kerry Blue Terrier, Manchester Terrier, Papillion, Pembroke Welsh Corgi, Poodle (all varieties)	?	MT	V	
von Willebrand's disease type 3	Scottish Terrier, Shetland Sheepdog	AR	MT	V	[45]
Parentage and individual identification	All breeds			VGL	

Abbreviations: AR, autosomal recessive; AD, autosomal dominant; LMT, linked marker test; MOI, mode of inheritance; ?, MOI not completely defined; MT, mutation test.

aPlease refer to Appendix for key and contact information for diagnostic test laboratories.

Table 2
Commercial tests available for inherited diseases and traits in cats as of August 31, 2005

Disease/trait	Breed	MOI	Type of test	Test laboratory[a]	References
Agouti (tabby versus solid)	All breeds	AD	MT	VGL	
Gangliosidosis 1, 2	Korats	AR	MT	A	
Glycogenosis type IV	Norwegian Forest Cat	AR	MT	P	[46]
Mannosidosis	Domestic long-haired and short-haired, Persian	AR	MT	P	[47]
Mucopolysaccharidosis VI	Siamese	AR	MT	P	[48,49]
Mucopolysaccharidosis VII	Domestic short-haired	AR	MT	P	[50]
Polycystic kidney disease	Exotic, Himalayan, Persian, Persian crosses	AD	MT	VGL, V	[51]
Pyruvate kinase deficiency	Abyssinian Domestic Short-haired, Somali	AR	MT	P	
Spinal muscular atrophy	Maine Coon	AR	MT	M	
Parentage and individual identification	All breeds			VGL	

Abbreviations: AR, autosomal recessive; AD, autosomal dominant; MOI, mode of inheritance; MT, mutation test.
[a]Please refer to Appendix for key and contact information for diagnostic test laboratories.

cloning of his or her pet. The cost of processing the biopsies varies from $395 up to $1500 in addition to the veterinarian's fees for obtaining the samples from up to eight different sites. Samples are then stored by the companies for approximately $100 per year. Veterinarians also provide care for the newly cloned pets for their clients. Currently, a cat clone can be obtained for $32,000. It is unclear how this might affect veterinary malpractice insurance, which is based on the replacement cost of the pet.

Cloning of domestic animals is an inefficient process. In the first successful cat cloning experiment, eight recipient cats were used to obtain one live clone. In the dog cloning experiment, the efficiency was even lower, with two live births (only one puppy survived beyond 3 weeks) from 123 canine recipients. A diagram of the cloning process is provided in Fig. 3. Poor cloning efficiency means that many recipient animals are used to create just one clone, which raises ethical concerns for the veterinarian and the client to consider.

Unfortunately, cloning is not at a point yet where an animal can be exactly duplicated. Although the genetic material is identical, there are epigenetic differences occurring in the developing embryo that are not recapitulated in clones [64,65]. Epigenetic change alters the phenotype (usually a change in gene expression) without a change in the DNA sequence. An obvious difference was seen in the first cloned cat. The animal that was cloned was a calico, and the clone was gray and white. The patches of color seen in calico and tortoiseshell cats are attributable to random inactivation of the X chromosome in female mammals. The orange coat color gene is located on the X chromosome, and because X inactivation occurs in a random fashion, the cats that carry one X

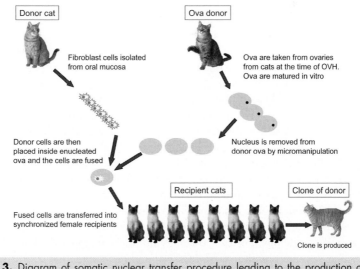

Fig. 3. Diagram of somatic nuclear transfer procedure leading to the production of a cat clone.

chromosome coding for orange and one coding for gray end up with patches of the two colors. The clone in this case no longer had random X inactivation. The somatic cell nuclei used to produce the clone must have had the X chromosome carrying the orange allele inactivated, and this was not reset by the cloning process. The only health manifestation of not having random X inactivation is that a female animal has effectively only one X chromosome, making it more susceptible to X-linked diseases similar to male animals.

There are other types of epigenetic modification that may not be accurately replicated in clones, including imprinting, which is the unequal expression of genes from the paternal and maternal genomes. Because clones are produced from differentiated cells, the marks that distinguish paternal from maternal genomes are different from those in an embryo. There are more than 45 genes that are known to be imprinted in mammals. Many of these genes are involved with growth and development of the embryo as well as the placenta. It is thought that the fetal overgrowth syndromes seen in some clones are caused by inappropriate imprinting of the IGFIIR gene [65]. Other imprinted genes may also play an important role in the abnormal development that occurs in many clones.

A third type of epigenetic modification that may play a role in the health of clones is telomere length. Reports that Dolly the sheep, the first cloned mammal, lived a shortened life and had early onset of arthritis have fueled studies into the aging process in cloned animals [66]. Telomeres are the sequences at the ends of the chromosomes. They protect the chromosome ends from degradation and allow efficient replication. Over time, the telomeres shorten; eventually, they become so short that DNA replication stops. Another type of epigenetic modification is the control of telomere length. Thus, telomere length may also be improperly regulated in clones in a tissue-specific manner [65].

The differences between clones and their "parents" that are likely to be most important to clients are the appearance and behavior of the clone. The coat pattern of calico or tortoiseshell cats is going to be different based on differences in the pattern of X inactivation in clones versus the original animal. Other coat patterns that have a stochastic influence might also be different. For example, the spot location on Dalmatians, the pattern of gray and black seen with the Merle locus in many herding breeds, and the location of the black stripes in Brindle-coated dogs may be different between clones and parents. Clients may be disappointed to find that the clone does not look exactly like the parent.

The behavior or temperament may be different in clones based on the environmental differences in the way that clones are raised. Many of the animals that people are interested in cloning are mixed breed and were adopted from a shelter. Their early environment is completely unknown. Clones are raised for the first 3 months in a laboratory environment, which is quite different from how the original animal was raised. In addition, clones are most likely to be raised as singletons. For cats, this may not make a large difference in personality, but puppies obtain important social and developmental cues from interacting with their littermates. Cloning is a complicated procedure, and the creation of an exact duplicate is not at all certain at this point in time.

SUMMARY

The state of genetic knowledge in dogs and cats is ever growing. The genes responsible for numerous diseases and traits in companion animals are known. Using this information, many screening and diagnostic genetic tests are available to assist veterinarians in providing more informed medical advice to clients. With sequencing of the dog and cat genomes, more knowledge and many more genetic tests will become available to the veterinary community in the coming years. Not only are these genetic insights likely to play a role in diagnosis and prevention of disease through selective breeding; they may also lead to clinically feasible gene therapies. Finally, cloning of cats and dogs is now possible, and it is, in part, the veterinarian's role to help clients understand the ramifications of the cloning process so that they can make an informed decision. Although not every veterinarian is expected to become an expert in the ever-changing field of veterinary genetics, hopefully, they should see that there is a wealth of genetic resources available with the goal of diagnosing, treating, and preventing disease in their patients.

APPENDIX

Test Laboratories

A: Auburn University (Auburn, Alabama)
H.J. Baker; Scott-Ritchey Research Center
Bakerhj@vetmed.auburn.edu
(334) 844-5951

H: HealthGene Corporation (Toronto, Ontario, Canada)
http://www.healthgene.com/canine/index.asp
(877) 371-1551

M: Michigan State University (East Lansing, Michigan)
Laboratory of Comparative Medical Genetics
http://mmg.msu.edu/faculty/fyfe.htm
fyfe@cvm.msu.edu

O: Optigen, LLC (Ithaca, New York)
http://www.optigen.com/
(607) 257-0301

P: PennGen Laboratories (Philadelphia, Pennsylvania)
http://w3.vet.upenn.edu/research/centers/penngen/
(215) 898-8894

V: VetGen (Ann Arbor, Michigan)
http://www.vetgen.com/
(800) 483-8436

VGL: Veterinary Genetics Laboratory (Davis, California)
http://www.vgl.ucdavis.edu/
(530) 752-2211

W: Washington State University (Pullman, Washington)
Veterinary Clinical Pharmacology Laboratory
http://www.vetmed.wsu.edu/depts-VCPL/
(509) 335-3745

References

[1] Henthorn PS, Somberg RL, Fimiani VM, et al. IL-2R gamma gene microdeletion demonstrates that canine X-linked severe combined immunodeficiency is a homologue of the human disease. Genomics 1994;23(1):69–74.

[2] Whitney KM, Goodman SA, Bailey EM, et al. The molecular basis of canine pyruvate kinase deficiency. Exp Hematol 1994;22(9):866–74.

[3] Ostrander EA, Lindblad-Toh K, Lander ES. Sequencing the genome of the domestic dog Canis familiaris. Available at: http://www.genome.gov/Pages/Research/Sequencing/SeqProposals/CanineSEQedited.pdf. Accessed August 16, 2005.

[4] O'Brien SJ, Lander ES, Haskins ME, et al. Sequencing the genome of the domestic cat Felis catus. Available at: http://www.genome.gov/Pages/Research/Sequencing/SeqProposals/CatSEQ.pdf. 2002. Accessed August 16, 2005.

[5] Metallinos DL. Canine molecular genetic testing. Vet Clin North Am Small Anim Pract 2001;31:421–31.

[6] Benson KF, Li FQ, Person RE, et al. Mutations associated with neutropenia in dogs and humans disrupt intracellular transport of neutrophil elastase. Nat Genet 2003;35(1):90–6.

[7] Victoria T, Rafi MA, Wenger DA. Cloning of the canine GALC cDNA and identification of the mutation causing globoid cell leukodystrophy in West Highland White and Cairn terriers. Genomics 1996;33(3):457–62.

[8] Debenham SL, Millington A, Kijast J, et al. Canine leucocyte adhesion deficiency in Irish red and white setters. J Small Anim Pract 2002;43(2):74–5.

[9] Kijas JM, Bauer TR Jr, Gafvert S, et al. A missense mutation in the beta-2 integrin gene (ITGB2) causes canine leukocyte adhesion deficiency. Genomics 1999;61(1):101–7.

[10] Sharp NJ, Kornegay JN, Van Camp SD, et al. An error in dystrophin mRNA processing in golden retriever muscular dystrophy, an animal homologue of Duchenne muscular dystrophy. Genomics 1992;13(1):115–21.

[11] He Q, Madsen M, Kilkenney A, et al. Amnionless function is required for cubilin brush-border expression and intrinsic factor-cobalamin (vitamin B12) absorption in vivo. Blood 2005;106(4):1447–53.

[12] Lowe JK, Kukekova AV, Kirkness EF, et al. Linkage mapping of the primary disease locus for collie eye anomaly. Genomics 2003;82(1):86–95.

[13] Bedford PG. Collie eye anomaly in the Lancashire heeler. Vet Rec 1998;143(13):354–6.

[14] Sidjanin DJ, Lowe JK, McElwee JL, et al. Canine CNGB3 mutations establish cone degeneration as orthologous to the human achromatopsia locus ACHM3. Hum Mol Genet 2002;11(16):1823–33.

[15] Fyfe JC, Kampschmidt K, Dang V, et al. Congenital hypothyroidism with goiter in toy fox terriers. J Vet Intern Med 2003;17(1):50–7.

[16] Aguirre GD, Baldwin V, Pearce-Kelling S, et al. Congenital stationary night blindness in the dog: common mutation in the RPE65 gene indicates founder effect. Mol Vis 1998;4:23–9.

[17] Yuzbasiyan-Gurkan V, Blanton SH, Cao Y, et al. Linkage of a microsatellite marker to the canine copper toxicosis locus in Bedlington terriers. Am J Vet Res 1997;58(1):23–7.

[18] van De Sluis B, Rothuizen J, Pearson PL, et al. Identification of a new copper metabolism gene by positional cloning in a purebred dog population. Hum Mol Genet 2002;11(2):165–73.

[19] Henthorn PS, Liu J, Gidalevich T, et al. Canine cystinuria: polymorphism in the canine SLC3A1 gene and identification of a nonsense mutation in cystinuric Newfoundland dogs. Hum Genet 2000;107(4):295–303.

[20] Skelly BJ, Sargan DR, Winchester BG, et al. Genomic screening for fucosidosis in English Springer Spaniels. Am J Vet Res 1999;60(6):726–9.

[21] Wang ZH, Zeng B, Shibuya H, et al. Isolation and characterization of the normal canine beta-galactosidase gene and its mutation in a dog model of GM1-gangliosidosis. J Inherit Metab Dis 2000;23(6):593–606.

[22] Brooks MB, Gu W, Ray K. Complete deletion of factor IX gene and inhibition of factor IX activity in a labrador retriever with hemophilia B. J Am Vet Med Assoc 1997;211(11): 1418–21.

[23] Mauser AE, Whitlark J, Whitney KM, et al. A deletion mutation causes hemophilia B in Lhasa Apso dogs. Blood 1996;88(9):3451–5.

[24] Ellinwood NM, Wang P, Skeen T, et al. A model of mucopolysaccharidosis IIIB (Sanfilippo syndrome type IIIB): N-acetyl-alpha-D-glucosaminidase deficiency in Schipperke dogs. J Inherit Metab Dis 2003;26(5):489–504.

[25] Ray J, Bouvet A, DeSanto C, et al. Cloning of the canine beta-glucuronidase cDNA, mutation identification in canine MPS VII, and retroviral vector-mediated correction of MPS VII cells. Genomics 1998;48(2):248–53.

[26] Mealey KL, Bentjen SA, Gay JM, et al. Ivermectin sensitivity in collies is associated with a deletion mutation of the mdr1 gene. Pharmacogenetics 2001;11(8):727–33.

[27] Rhodes TH, Vite CH, Giger U, et al. A missense mutation in canine C1C-1 causes recessive myotonia congenita in the dog. FEBS Lett 1999;456(1):54–8.

[28] Bhalerao DP, Rajpurohit Y, Vite CH, et al. Detection of a genetic mutation for myotonia congenita among Miniature Schnauzers and identification of a common carrier ancestor. Am J Vet Res 2002;63(10):1443–7.

[29] Hungs M, Fan J, Lin L, et al. Identification and functional analysis of mutations in the hypocretin (orexin) genes of narcoleptic canines. Genome Res 2001;11(4):531–9.

[30] Lin L, Faraco J, Li R, et al. The sleep disorder canine narcolepsy is caused by a mutation in the hypocretin (orexin) receptor 2 gene. Cell 1999;98(3):365–76.

[31] Melville SA, Wilson CL, Chiang CS, et al. A mutation in canine CLN5 causes neuronal ceroid lipofuscinosis in Border collie dogs. Genomics 2005;86(3):287–94.

[32] Giger U, Smith BF, Woods CB, et al. Inherited phosphofructokinase deficiency in an American cocker spaniel. J Am Vet Med Assoc 1992;201(10):1569–71.

[33] Smith BF, Stedman H, Rajpurohit Y, et al. Molecular basis of canine muscle type phosphofructokinase deficiency. J Biol Chem 1996;271(33):20070–4.

[34] Kijas JW, Cideciyan AV, Aleman TS, et al. Naturally occurring rhodopsin mutation in the dog causes retinal dysfunction and degeneration mimicking human dominant retinitis pigmentosa. Proc Natl Acad Sci USA 2002;99(9):6328–33.

[35] Suber ML, Pittler SJ, Qin N, et al. Irish setter dogs affected with rod/cone dysplasia contain a nonsense mutation in the rod cGMP phosphodiesterase beta-subunit gene. Proc Natl Acad Sci USA 1993;90(9):3968–72.

[36] Ray K, Baldwin VJ, Acland GM, et al. Cosegregation of codon 807 mutation of the canine rod cGMP phosphodiesterase beta gene and rcd1. Invest Ophthalmol Vis Sci 1994;35(13): 4291–9.

[37] Ray K, Tejero MD, Baldwin VJ, et al. An improved diagnostic test for rod cone dysplasia 1 (rcd1) using allele-specific polymerase chain reaction. Curr Eye Res 1996;15(5):583–7.

[38] Dekomien G, Runte M, Godde R, et al. Generalized progressive retinal atrophy of Sloughi dogs is due to an 8-bp insertion in exon 21 of the PDE6B gene. Cytogenet Cell Genet 2000;90(3–4):261–7.

[39] Petersen-Jones SM, Entz DD, Sargan DR. cGMP phosphodiesterase-alpha mutation causes progressive retinal atrophy in the Cardigan Welsh corgi dog. Invest Ophthalmol Vis Sci 1999;40(8):1637–44.

[40] Petersen-Jones SM, Zhu FX. Development and use of a polymerase chain reaction-based diagnostic test for the causal mutation of progressive retinal atrophy in Cardigan Welsh Corgis. Am J Vet Res 2000;61(7):844–6.

[41] Whitney KM, Lothrop CD Jr. Genetic test for pyruvate kinase deficiency of Basenjis. J Am Vet Med Assoc 1995;207(7):918–21.

[42] Giger U, Mason GD, Wang P. Inherited erythrocyte pyruvate kinase deficiency in a beagle dog. Vet Clin Pathol 1991;20(3):83–6.

[43] Skelly BJ, Wallace M, Rajpurohit YR, et al. Identification of a 6 base pair insertion in West Highland White Terriers with erythrocyte pyruvate kinase deficiency. Am J Vet Res 1999;60(9):1169–72.

[44] Pullen RP, Somberg RL, Felsburg PJ, et al. X-linked severe combined immunodeficiency in a family of Cardigan Welsh corgis. J Am Anim Hosp Assoc 1997;33(6):494–9.

[45] Venta PJ, Li J, Yuzbasiyan-Gurkan V, et al. Mutation causing von Willebrand's disease in Scottish Terriers. J Vet Intern Med 2000;14(1):10–9.

[46] Fyfe JC, Giger U, Van Winkle TJ, et al. Glycogen storage disease type IV: inherited deficiency of branching enzyme activity in cats. Pediatr Res 1992;32(6):719–25.

[47] Berg T, Tollersrud OK, Walkley SU, et al. Purification of feline lysosomal alpha-mannosidase, determination of its cDNA sequence and identification of a mutation causing alpha-mannosidosis in Persian cats. Biochem J 1997;328(Pt 3):863–70.

[48] Yogalingam G, Litjens T, Bielicki J, et al. Feline mucopolysaccharidosis type VI. Characterization of recombinant N-acetylgalactosamine 4-sulfatase and identification of a mutation causing the disease. J Biol Chem 1996;271(44):27259–65.

[49] Crawley AC, Muntz FH, Haskins ME, et al. Prevalence of mucopolysaccharidosis type VI mutations in Siamese cats. J Vet Intern Med 2003;17(4):495–8.

[50] Fyfe JC, Kurzhals RL, Lassaline ME, et al. Molecular basis of feline beta-glucuronidase deficiency: an animal model of mucopolysaccharidosis VII. Genomics 1999;58(2):121–8.

[51] Lyons LA, Biller DS, Erdman CA, et al. Feline polycystic kidney disease mutation identified in PKD1. J Am Soc Nephrol 2004;15(10):2548–55.

[52] Kay MA, Rothenberg S, Landen CN, et al. In vivo gene therapy of hemophilia B: sustained partial correction in factor IX-deficient dogs. Science 1993;262(5130):117–9.

[53] Wang L, Herzog RW. AAV-mediated gene transfer for treatment of hemophilia. Curr Gene Ther 2005;5(3):349–60.

[54] Acland GM, Aguirre GD, Ray J, et al. Gene therapy restores vision in a canine model of childhood blindness. Nat Genet 2001;28(1):92–5.

[55] Narfstrom K, Katz ML, Ford M, et al. In vivo gene therapy in young and adult RPE65−/− dogs produces long-term visual improvement. J Hered 2003;94(1):31–7.

[56] Yanay O, Barry SC, Katen LJ, et al. Treatment of canine cyclic neutropenia by lentivirus-mediated G-CSF delivery. Blood 2003;102(6):2046–52.

[57] Vite CH, McGowan JC, Niogi SN, et al. Effective gene therapy for an inherited CNS disease in a large animal model. Ann Neurol 2005;57(3):355–64.

[58] Ponder KP, Melniczek JR, Xu L, et al. Therapeutic neonatal hepatic gene therapy in mucopolysaccharidosis VII dogs. Proc Natl Acad Sci USA 2002;99(20):13102–7.

[59] Choi EW, Shin IS, Youn HY, et al. Gene therapy using non-viral peptide vector in a canine systemic lupus erythematosus model. Vet Immunol Immunopathol 2005;103(3–4):223–33.

[60] Shin T, Kraemer D, Pryor J, et al. A cat cloned by nuclear transplantation. Nature 2002; 415(6874):859.

[61] Yin XJ, Lee HS, Lee YH, et al. Cats cloned from fetal and adult somatic cells by nuclear transfer. Reproduction 2005;129(2):245–9.

[62] Gomez MC, Pope CE, Giraldo A, et al. Birth of African Wildcat cloned kittens born from domestic cats. Cloning Stem Cells 2004;6(3):247–58.

[63] Lee BC, Kim MK, Jang G, et al. Dogs cloned from adult somatic cells. Nature 2005; 436(7051):641.

[64] Hiiragi T, Solter D. Reprogramming is essential in nuclear transfer. Mol Reprod Dev 2005;70(4):417–21.

[65] Shi W, Zakhartchenko V, Wolf E. Epigenetic reprogramming in mammalian nuclear transfer. Differentiation 2003;71(2):91–113.

[66] Adam D. Clone pioneer calls for health tests. Nature 2002;415(6868):103.

Vet Clin Small Anim 36 (2006) 475–501

VETERINARY CLINICS
SMALL ANIMAL PRACTICE

ELSEVIER
SAUNDERS

Pediatric Neurology of the Dog and Cat

James A. Lavely, DVM

The Animal Care Center, 6470 Redwood Drive, Rohnert Park, CA 94928, USA

The neurologic examination in the puppy or kitten can be a challenging experience. Uncooperative patients, nervous system development, environmental stimuli, and the brief life experience of pediatric patients make a puppy or kitten's examination unique, thus complicating the examination and its interpretation. Understanding the development of behavior reflexes and movement in puppies and kittens enables us to overcome some of these challenges and to recognize the neurologically abnormal patient. Subsequently, we can identify the neuroanatomic localization and generate a differential diagnosis list. This article first reviews the pediatric neurologic examination and then discusses diseases unique to these individuals.

Signalment and a thorough history are the first part of any examination. Information regarding problematic parturition, affected littermates, health of the parents, feline leukemia virus (FeLV) and feline immunodeficiency virus (FIV) status, nutrition, and vaccination history should be obtained. Time of onset of signs as well as their progression may help to rule in or rule out inherited, developmental, and acquired disorders. Identifying where the patient was obtained may be helpful, because certain animal shelters or regions may have a high incidence of distemper or panleukopenia. Catteries may have a high incidence of feline infectious peritonitis (FIP).

NEUROLOGIC DEVELOPMENT
Mental Status
The main activities of puppies and kittens during the first 2 weeks of life are sleeping and nursing [1,2]. Puppies do not usually sleep alone until approximately 5 to 6 weeks of age [3]. Kittens may display considerable motor activity during sleep in the first week [2]. Kittens transition directly from waking into rapid eye movement (REM) sleep [4]. During periods of sleep, puppies and kittens can be roused [2,5]. Initially, an electroencephalographic (EEG) scan of the neonatal puppy is similar during periods of sleep and waking [5]. EEG patterns are of low amplitude and irregular for the first week of life. During the second week, patterns become more regular and increase in amplitude and frequency.

E-mail address: jim_lavely@yahoo.com

0195-5616/06/$ – see front matter
doi:10.1016/j.cvsm.2005.12.009

A reduction in neonatal spindles is seen on EEG scans [6]. EEG differences between sleeping and waking develop at approximately 3 weeks of age [5]. An increase in amplitude and decrease in frequency of slow waves as well as increasing fast activity are seen during an alert EEG scan [6]. All phases of EEG activity seen during alert, drowsy, paroxysmal sleep, quiet sleep, and activated sleep (REM) are present by the fourth and fifth weeks. In general, the EEG pattern increases in amplitude until 7 weeks of age [7]. Adult-like EEG patterns develop at 8 weeks of age [5].

Gait and Posture

Vestibular function is present at birth and is important for positioning during nursing. Muscular coordination, however, is lacking [1]. Initial movements are characterized by swimming-like movements of the limbs while sliding along on the ventral abdomen and thorax [7]. The ability to raise the head is present at birth in puppies and kittens, and the head may be used initially to right oneself (righting reflex) [2,5]. An upright posture in puppies cannot be maintained until 10 to 14 days of age [5]. At birth, the body posture is primarily one of flexion. If suspended by the head, flexor hypertonicity is present (Fig. 1). At 4 to 5 days of age in puppies, the flexor hypertonicity is replaced by extension (Fig. 2) until 3 to 4 weeks of age, when the puppy struggles to escape when held in suspension [7]. Timing of extensor dominance is much more variable in kittens [8]. By 5 to

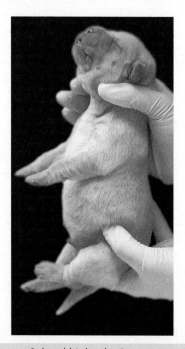

Fig. 1. Flexor dominance in a 2-day-old Labrador Retriever puppy. Note that the thoracic limbs are primarily in flexion.

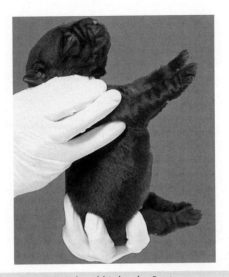

Fig. 2. Extensor dominance in a 5-day-old Labrador Retriever puppy. Note the extension in the thoracic limbs.

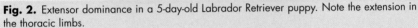

6 days of age, puppies supported in the thoracic limbs can make stepping movements. The pelvic limbs do not make meaningful stepping movements until 7 to 10 days of age. At 14 to 16 days of age, the pelvic limbs begin to support body weight [7]. Timing to support weight is similar in kittens [2]. An uncoordinated gait begins at 18 to 21 days of age [1]. Adult postural and balancing abilities develop between 6 and 8 weeks of age [5]. Breed variation does exist, because Greyhound puppies can raise themselves by the pelvic limbs at 1 day of age, whereas Dachshunds cannot do so for several days [5].

Tactile placing reactions in puppies can be seen in the thoracic limbs between 2 and 4 days of age and in the pelvic limbs between 5 and 9 days of age [3]. Other reports cite that tactile placing does not develop until the second to third week, with the thoracic limb reactions developing before those of the pelvic limbs [5, 7]. By 5 weeks of age, tactile placing responses are more consistent. Hopping reactions are difficult to elicit until 6 to 8 weeks of age [5]. Hopping reactions are present in the thoracic limbs before the pelvic limbs [7]. Extensor postural thrust can be seen by days 12 to 14 in puppies [9] and days 14 to 16 in kittens [2] (Figs. 3 and 4).

Tonic neck reflexes (magnus reflex) evaluate tension receptors in the cervical region and can be obtained as soon as 1 day of age in the dog. The reflexes become more obvious after 5 to 6 days and are more vigorous in the thoracic limbs compared with the pelvic limbs. Extension of the neck results in extension of the thoracic limbs and flexion of the pelvic limbs. Flexion of the neck results in extension of the pelvic limbs. Lateral flexion of the neck results in extension of the ipsilateral limb and flexion of the contralateral limb [7]. Kittens continuously inhibit these reflexes, and if present beyond 3 weeks of age, an

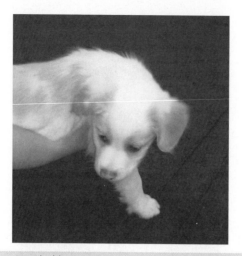

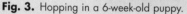

Fig. 3. Hopping in a 6-week-old puppy.

upper motor neuron lesion is indicated [2]. In one study, a magnus reflex could not be obtained in any of 22 kittens [8].

A "diving" reflex can be identified at 3 weeks of age when the puppy is held horizontally under the chest and is rocked backward or forward. The puppy extends its thoracic limbs, raises its head, and arches its back [5]. Also, at 3 weeks, a "seal" reflex develops, where if suspended under the ventral thorax, an extension of the head with pelvic limb extension and flexion or extension of the thoracic limbs results [7].

Normal responses to being dropped are seen at 3 to 4 weeks of age. The animal twists the head, neck, and trunk into an upright position while extending all limbs in anticipation of impact [2,5].

Cranial Nerves

Reflexes to protect the eyes develop before the eyes actually open. A blink reflex (cranial nerves [CNs] II and VII) secondary to light stimulation occurs within 24 to 48 hours of birth [2,3,5,7]. Interestingly, this is also before development of the retina. Electroretinographic (ERG) activity at this time is absent in the puppy [7]. The pupillary light reflex (CNs II and III) is present when the eyes open at 10 to 16 days of age in the puppy [7] and at 5 to 14 days of age in the kitten [2]. Pupillary response is usually slow and likely corresponds to the developing retina [3,7,10]. In the puppy, the a-wave of the ERG pattern is negative at 10 days and matures greatly over the next week. The b-wave is present by day 15 and is well developed by day 21. At 28 days of age, the ERG pattern is that of an adult. At this time, pupillary light reflexes are similar to those of an adult [7]. The menace response may be present but slow when the eyes open. This response may not be present until 3 to 4 weeks of age [1,2].

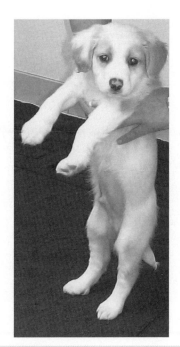

Fig. 4. Extensor postural thrust in a 6-week-old puppy.

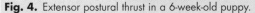

In puppies, the vibrissopalpebral reflex (CNs V and VII) is present at 1 to 2 days of age [5]. Palpebral reflexes (CNs V and VII) develop within 2 to 4 days of birth in the puppy and within 1 to 3 days in the kitten [3,10]. The corneal reflex in puppies (CNs V and VI) develops as soon as the eyes open [3,7]. The corneal reflex continues to mature until approximately 5 weeks of age. Physiologic nystagmus (CNs III, IV, VI, and VIII) is present on opening of the eyelids [7]. Kittens may demonstrate a divergent strabismus until 8 weeks of age [2].

The structures of the middle and inner ear are well differentiated at birth. The external ear canals open between 12 and 14 days of age in puppies [3,7] and between 6 and 14 days in kittens [2]. At this time, a brisk startle response (CN VIII) can be produced with auditory stimulation [3]. Auditory evoked potentials are first recordable at this time and are relatively mature in the puppy at 3 to 4 weeks of age [7] and at 4 to 5 weeks of age in the kitten [11,12].

Olfaction (CN I) is present at birth but is likely poorly developed [1]. The swallowing reflex (CNs IX and X) is present soon after parturition. The suckling reflex (CNs V, VII, and XII) is present within 1 to 2 days of age (Fig. 5) [5]. The suckling reflex disappears by 20 days in the kitten [13]. The hypoglossal nerve (CN XII) can be further evaluated by examining tongue size and symmetry. The rooting reflex is tested by cupping the fingers around the muzzle. This

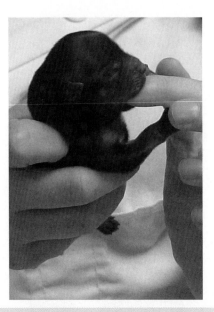

Fig. 5. Suckling reflex in a 1- to 2-hour-old newborn puppy.

stimulates the puppy to "root" or push forward and is strongest during the first 2 weeks, before it disappears at approximately 25 days (Table 1) [1].

Spinal and Myotactic Reflexes

The patellar, triceps, gastrocnemius, withdrawal, and panniculus reflexes are all present shortly after birth but may be difficult to elicit [5,7]. These reflexes become more helpful once the period of hypertonicity abates [7]. A crossed extensor reflex is normally present shortly after birth. If the crossed extensor reflex persists past 17 days in the kitten or past 3 weeks of age in the puppy, however, it is indicative of an upper motor neuron lesion, representing a loss of

Table 1 Time to onset of positive cranial nerve tests		
Reflex	Puppy	Kitten
PLR	10–16 d	5–14 d
Dazzle	1–2 d	1–2 d
Palpebral	2–4 d	1–3 d
Menace response	10 d–4 w	1–4 w
Corneal	10–16 d	5–14 d
Vibrissopalpebral	1–2 d	
Suckling	1–2 d	1–2 d

Abbreviations: d, days; PLR, pupillary light reflex; w, weeks.

contralateral inhibition [2,3,7]. The loss of the crossed extensor reflex may be correlated to myelinization [14]. Stimulation of the superficial anal, preputial, or vulval reflex causes excretory behavior shortly after birth [5]. Generally, reflex urination cannot be elicited after 3 weeks [14]. It may persist throughout the juvenile period as a submissive response, however [5]. When testing spinal reflexes, it is important to have the patient as relaxed as possible and in lateral recumbency. This diminishes the hypertonicity that can be present in other body positions.

A response to pinprick pain (eg, vocalization) can be obtained in the newborn puppy and kitten [7,10].

Nervous System Maturation

Histologic examination of the canine spinal cord indicates that maturity is reached at 6 weeks of age. The fasciculus gracilis and lateral corticospinal tract are the last to become myelinated. Initially, the ventral columns have greater myelination compared with the dorsal columns. With increasing age, the dorsal column fibers become larger than the ventral column fibers. Lateral fibers seem to be the slowest to mature and may do so after 6 weeks of age. The cranial aspect of the spinal cord tends to develop slightly sooner than the caudal portion [14].

Feline maturation occurs sooner than maturation in the dog. The lateral columns are well myelinated by 14 days of age. The corticospinal and rubrospinal fibers are still poorly myelinated at 35 days, however. The ventral columns may be well myelinated as early as 8 days of age. These findings may explain the slightly quicker clinical development in cats compared with dogs [14].

Nervous system maturation also affects nerve conduction testing. Sciatic-tibial and ulnar nerve conduction velocity (NCV) is approximately half of adult values. Adult NCV is reached between 6 months and 1 year of age. Kittens reach adult NCV values at 3 months of age. This corresponds with the time when nerve fiber diameter reaches adult values. Given the correlation in kittens and people, it is suspected that axonal diameter reaches maturity between 6 months and 1 year in the dog [15].

During maturation, response to injury may be greater than in the adult. Puppies less than 8 weeks of age experiencing spinal cord transection may develop the ability to spinal walk within 2 months. This response is characterized by an alternating nonpropulsive pelvic limb stride without correlation to the thoracic limb stride. Adults experiencing thoracolumbar transection typically require several months to develop spinal walking [7]. Further evidence supporting a diagnosis of spinal walking is urinary incontinence and the lack of apparent deep pain sensation.

It is important to rule out metabolic causes for diffuse brain signs or seizures in the neonatal puppy or kitten. Neonates withheld adequate nutrition may be hypoglycemic or have a compromised immune system, and therefore may be more likely to develop infections. Portosystemic shunts may cause altered mentation and/or seizures. Additionally, certain breed-related conditions or anomalies should be considered.

INFECTIOUS DISEASE
Distemper
Canine distemper virus (CDV) is a single-stranded RNA morbillivirus closely related to the measles virus. CDV is typically transmitted through an aerosol route, first infecting the upper respiratory system. Primary viral replication occurs in lymphoid tissues. Immunosuppression results, with T cells affected predominantly [16]. CDV is epitheliotropic, spreading to the respiratory system, central nervous system (CNS), intestinal tract, integument, and urinary bladder [16,17]. CDV enters the CNS through the cerebrospinal fluid (CSF) or crosses the blood-brain barrier via infected mononuclear cells [16,18]. CDV infection results in multifocal CNS lesions affecting white and gray matter. White matter is more often affected, where primary demyelination occurs. Predilection sites include the cerebellum, periventricular white matter, optic pathways, and spinal cord [16].

Dogs less than 1 year of age are typically affected, although persistent viral infection may also lead to chronic or "old dog distemper." Outbreaks may be seen, particularly at animal shelters, because of diverse populations, crowded conditions, and stress favoring transmission. Vaccination has decreased the incidence of distemper; however, 30% of distemper cases occur in vaccinated dogs [18]. Neurologic signs are often focal, despite multifocal lesions. Seizures and myoclonus are the most commonly reported neurologic abnormalities. Caudal fossa and myelopathic signs are also reported [19]. The cause for CDV-induced myoclonus is uncertain; however, hyperexcitability of the lower motor neuron is suspected. The myoclonus may persist during sleep but is abolished with anesthesia [20].

Extraneural signs are common, reflecting a high incidence of pneumonia, conjunctivitis, rhinitis, and enteritis. Hyperkeratosis of the nasal planum and foot pads may also occur. Affected dogs may also have discolored teeth because of enamel hypoplasia [18,19].

The diagnosis of distemper is often based on clinical signs. CDV should be highly suspected when neurologic signs, particularly myoclonus, are present in combination with respiratory signs in a young dog. Thoracic radiographs frequently identify pulmonary infiltrates [19]. CSF analysis often yields a mononuclear pleocytosis but may also be normal, and, less commonly, albuminocytologic dissociation is identified [18]. Serologic detection is not extremely useful, because high CDV titers may be secondary to prior vaccination or previous subclinical infection. Furthermore, severe CDV infections may result in a low titer because of strong immunosuppression. Direct immunofluorescence testing of conjunctival, nasal, and vaginal smears can confirm CDV only within 3 weeks of infection [17]. Reverse transcriptase polymerase chain reaction (RT-PCR) is thought to be the best antemortem method used to detect CDV. RT-PCR detected CDV RNA in 86% of infected dogs via serum testing and in 88%

via CSF or whole-blood testing. Twenty-two of 22 dogs tested positive when using RT-PCR to evaluate urine. Twelve asymptomatic dogs tested negative using the same technique. It is unclear if these dogs had been vaccinated previously, however. Vaccine virus can be detected in urine a couple of days after vaccination [21]. Another study suggests that nested PCR may be more sensitive than single RT-PCR [17].

The prognosis for distemper infections is variable. Severely affected dogs are likely to succumb to the disease, whereas mildly affected dogs may recover. Therapy is supportive. Anticonvulsant therapy and antibiotics for pneumonia should be used as indicated. *Toxoplasma gondii* has been associated with CDV-infected dogs; if detected, a course of clindamycin is recommended [22].

Neosporosis

Neospora caninum is a primary CNS and neuromuscular pathogen. Pneumonia, myocarditis, hepatitis, myonecrosis, and encephalitis are the predominant lesions in neonatal infections. Ninety-two percent of affected dogs are less than 1 year of age. Transplacental transmission is the main route of infection. Ten percent of reported puppies died within 3 weeks of age. Puppies are typically presented for an ascending paraparesis. Signs may progress to the cervical, brain stem, and cerebellar regions. Pelvic limb hyperextension may be seen when polyradiculoneuritis or polymyositis is present. Creatine kinase may be elevated with polymyositis. CSF typically indicates a mononuclear pleocytosis. Serum immunofluorescence antibody (IFA) titers in affected dogs are greater than 1:200, although clinically normal dogs have had titers greater than 1:800. Tachyzoites may be found within cells obtained from CSF, bronchial lavage, and dermal lesions [23]. Clindamycin is the recommended antibiotic therapy [22], although trimethoprim-sulfadiazine may also be used [23]. The prognosis for neosporosis is poor [23]. Naturally occurring neosporosis has not been reported in cats.

Toxoplasmosis

Cats are the definitive host for *T gondii*. Transplacental infection in kittens causes the most severe clinical signs. Kittens may be stillborn or may die before weaning. Pulmonary, CNS, hepatic, pancreatic, cardiac, and ocular infections are commonly found in clinically infected cats [22,24]. Muscle involvement is not a significant feature in infected cats [25]. Despite the presence of microscopic brain abnormalities in 53 of 55 histologically examined cats, neurologic signs were only reported in 7 of 100 infected cats in one study. *Toxoplasma* organisms were identified in 80% of the examined brains. Disseminated glial-histiocytic granulomas were the most common histologic finding, along with mononuclear perivascular cuffing [24]. Most clinical cases are seen in cats older than 3 months of age and are associated with reactivated infection [22,25]. Serology may be used to identify IgM and IgG antibodies. Thirty percent of cats and dogs have *T gondii* antibodies, however [22,26]. CSF analysis in CNS toxoplasmosis typically causes a mixed pleocytosis with increased CSF protein. Clindamycin is considered the treatment of choice [22].

CONGENITAL AND DEVELOPMENTAL DISORDERS

Cerebellar Hypoplasia

Cerebellar hypoplasia commonly affects kittens. The disorder is typically secondary to in utero or perinatal infection with feline panleukopenia virus [27–29]. Affected kittens show signs of cerebellar disease, such as ataxia, hypermetria, and tremors, around 2 to 4 weeks of age. The virus affects the external germinal layer of the cerebellum, which develops until 10 weeks of age in dogs and cats. The development of the granule layer is disrupted, and the virus is cytopathic to Purkinje cells [28].

Cerebellar hypoplasia is most likely inherited in dogs. It has been reported in Wire-Haired Fox Terriers, Irish Terriers, and Chow Chows [27]. Parvovirus is not commonly considered to cause cerebellar hypoplasia in puppies. Parvovirus was isolated from two Blue Tick Coonhound littermates with cerebellar hypoplasia, however, indicating the potential to cause similar disease as in kittens [28]. Neonatal cerebellar ataxia has been reported in Coton de Tulear dogs. Ultrastructural evidence suggests a synaptic dysfunction, and histopathologic abnormalities were lacking [27]. Agenesis or hypoplasia of the cerebellar vermis has also been described in several breeds [30].

Cerebellar abiotrophies also result from degeneration of the Purkinje cells. Signs occur several weeks later than those of cerebellar hypoplasia, however [29]. Furthermore, clinical signs of cerebellar hypoplasia tend to remain static, whereas abiotrophies are progressive.

Hydrocephalus

CSF is produced from the choroid plexus of the lateral, third, and fourth ventricles and the subarachnoid space. CSF flows from the ventricular system to the subarachnoid space via the lateral apertures of the fourth ventricle. It is produced at a constant rate of 0.047 mL/min in the dog and 0.017 mL/min in the cat. Production is not affected by CSF pressure within the ventricular system but may slow if there is choroid plexus atrophy. CSF is largely absorbed in the arachnoid villus in a venous sinus or cerebral vein. CSF is also absorbed by the veins and lymphatics around spinal nerves and CNs [31].

Hydrocephalus is an increase in CSF volume and is a common congenital disorder in toy and brachiocephalic dogs [31]. Stenosis of the mesencephalic aqueduct is the most common malformation and often results in fusion of the rostral colliculi [32]. CSF accumulates rostral to the obstruction, and progressive cerebral cortical atrophy occurs. The ventricular system dilates and may result in tearing of ependymal cells and periventricular diverticula formation [33]. Most cases of hydrocephalus are asymptomatic, and ventriculomegaly is a common incidental finding in toy and brachiocephalic breeds [34]. Siamese cats may develop hydrocephalus from transmission of a hereditary autosomal recessive trait. FIP also causes hydrocephalus in cats [2].

Clinical signs of hydrocephalus are secondary to loss of cortical neurons or neuronal function, alterations in intracranial pressure, or periventricular edema secondary to abnormal CSF flows across ventricular walls. Clinical signs are referable to the anatomic location most affected. Cerebral, vestibular, and cerebellar signs may be seen. A ventral and/or lateral strabismus may be present because of a skull or orbit deformity or increased pressure on the mesencephalic tegmentum. Affected puppies often have a persistent fontanelle and a dome-shaped appearance to the head [35]. Changes in cerebral vascularity, a thinned calvarium, and decreased cerebral tissue may cause hydrocephalic dogs to be more sensitive to head trauma. The resulting hemorrhage may cause acute neurologic deterioration. Chronic subdural hematomas have been identified in a hydrocephalic dog [36].

Diagnosis may be obtained by MRI or CT (Fig. 6). If a fontanelle is persistent, ultrasound can be used to confirm the presence of hydrocephalus. MRI provides the most detailed evaluation of the disorder and allows superior evaluation of the ventricular system and brain stem [35]. MRI may also help to rule out underlying causes or concurrent hemorrhage. Hydrocephalus secondary to leiomyosarcoma was reported in a 2-month-old Chihuahua [37]. CSF analysis helps to rule out underlying inflammatory or infectious causes for hydrocephalus.

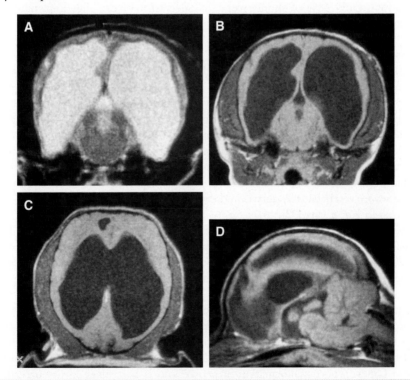

Fig. 6. Hydrocephalus. (A) Transverse T2-weighted image at the level of the midbrain. Note the dilated lateral ventricles. (B) Transverse T1-weighted image. (C) Dorsal plane image. The lateral ventricles are severely enlarged, with little remaining brain tissue. (D) Sagittal T1-weighted image.

Several medications have been shown to decrease CSF production and may be beneficial in symptomatic dogs. A slowly tapering course of prednisone starting at 0.5 mg/kg administered orally twice daily is often used. Glucocorticoids decrease CSF production by decreasing Na-K-ATPase activity [38] and also may have a beneficial effect on periventricular edema. Omeprazole also decreases CSF production, although its action may be independent of Na-K-ATPase inhibition [39]. Acetazolamide, a carbonic anhydrase inhibitor, may be used at 10 mg/kg administered orally every 6 to 8 hours. Potassium depletion may occur with use of acetazolamide, and electrolytes should be monitored [35].

Surgical therapy via ventriculoperitoneal shunting may be used to treat dogs with progressive signs nonresponsive to medical therapy. Shunts have not been proven more effective than medical therapy but do offer the possibility of long-term control of clinical signs [35]. One report claims fair to good success with the use of ventriculoperitoneal shunting [40]. Complications of shunt procedures include infection and undershunting because of blockage of the shunt [35]. A study of hydrocephalic children reported shunt failure in 177 of 344 children. Only 48% of shunts were still successful 1 year after implantation. Shunt obstruction was the most common cause of failure [41].

Lissencephaly

Lissencephaly is a congenital abnormality thought to arise from the arrest of neuronal migration to the cortical plate during fetal development. The aberrant development results in a smooth cortical surface without the development of gyri and sulci. The cerebral cortex is much thicker than normal. The corpus callosum and internal capsule fuse, resulting in the absence of a corona radiata [32,42]. Most cases of lissencephaly have been reported in the Lhasa Apso breed [32,42–44]. Lissencephaly has also been identified in a litter of Wire-Haired Fox Terriers. A litter of Irish Setters was reported to have lissencephaly and severe cerebellar hypoplasia and dysplasia. Lissencephaly has also been reported in Korat cats [32].

Clinical signs typically include seizures starting as early as 1 year of age. Visual deficits, obtundation, circling, and behavior changes may also occur [32,42,44]. These abnormalities may be identified in a puppy [44]. MRI identifies the loss of gyri and sulci as well as the thickened cortex (Fig. 7) [42].

Caudal Occipital Malformation Syndrome

Occipital bone hypoplasia leads to overcrowding of the caudal fossa and obstruction of the foramen magnum. This often results in syringohydromyelia of the cervical and, sometimes, thoracic spinal cord. The condition is similar to a Chiari type I malformation in people and is hereditary in the Cavalier King Charles Spaniel [45]. Caudal occipital hypoplasia has also been identified in the Maltese, Yorkshire Terrier, and Pomeranian [46]. Clinical signs are referable to a central cord syndrome and include persistent scratching at the cervical and/or shoulder region (particularly while on a leash), thoracic limb

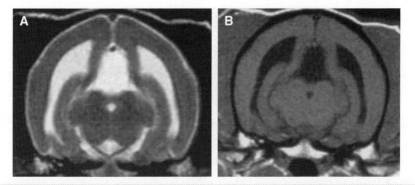

Fig. 7. Lissencephaly in a Lhasa Apso. Note the absence of gyri and sulci, giving the cerebral cortex a smooth appearance. (A) T2-weighted image. (B) T1-weighted image. (Courtesy of Gregg Kortz, DVM, Roseville, CA.)

weakness, cervical scoliosis, and pelvic limb ataxia. Some dogs may scream in apparent pain with a change in head position, excitement, or being touched in the paraesthetic region [45,47]. One report identified a significant number of dogs with facial nerve deficits, seizures, and vestibular signs [48]. Clinical signs typically occur between 6 months and 3 years of age; however, they have been identified as late as 10 years of age [45,49].

The pathophysiology of syringohydromyelia formation is not well understood. Syrinx formation results from abnormal CSF dynamics, with several theories as to the exact mechanism being postulated [47,50]. Cine MRI has confirmed abnormal or turbulent CSF flow in affected Cavalier King Charles Spaniels [51]. Damage to the dorsal horn in syringomyelia and alteration in substance P expression likely result in chronic pain [52].

Diagnosis is made via MRI of the brain and cervical spinal cord. MRI features include crowding of the caudal fossa, with caudal displacement of the cerebellum through the foramen magnum. The concurrent syringohydromyelia is hyperintense on T2 imaging and hypointense on T1 imaging (Fig. 8). A significant number of clinically normal Cavalier King Charles Spaniels may have MRI evidence of malformation [52].

Several medical treatment options may be tried with varying success. Prednisone can reduce inflammation that may be present near the syrinx, reduce pain, and possibly reduce CSF formation. Gabapentin may have a beneficial neuromodulatory effect. Proton pump inhibitors, such as omeprazole, can decrease CSF production, and therefore may be helpful [52].

Surgical therapy is recommended for patients with neurologic deterioration or significant pain and those refractory to medical therapy. The most common surgical approach is a suboccipital craniectomy with a dorsal laminectomy of C1. A durotomy may be done to relieve potential obstruction of CSF flow further [40,52,53]. Results of decompressive surgery are variable. In one study, none of 4 dogs improved after surgery [53], whereas in another study, 7 of

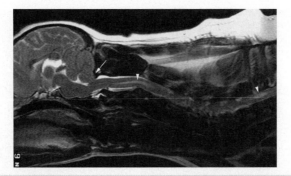

Fig. 8. Sagittal T2-weighted image reveals a Chiari malformation in a 4-year-old Cavalier King Charles Spaniel. The arrow denotes protrusion of the cerebellum through the foramen magnum. Syringohydromyelia is identified in the cervical and cranial thoracic spinal cord (*arrowheads*). (Courtesy of Heather Galano, DVM, Rohnert Park, CA.)

16 dogs achieved clinical resolution with decompressive surgery and another 6 of 16 dogs showed clinical improvement, for an overall success rate of 81.25%. Repeat surgery was required in 25% of these dogs because of constrictive scar tissue formation [46]. Repeat MRI in dogs after surgery often shows persistence of syringohydromyelia. It is generally thought that surgical intervention is most successful when signs are less severe and of shorter duration [52].

Atlantoaxial Instability

Atlantoaxial instability arises from aplasia, hypoplasia, or degeneration of the dens or associated ligaments leading to dorsal deviation of the dens [54,55]. Trauma may precipitate clinical signs in malformed dogs or may directly result in instability. Immature toy-breed dogs are typically affected, with the Yorkshire Terrier and Poodle overrepresented. Seventy percent of affected dogs are less than 1 year of age. Atlantoaxial instability leads to compression of the cranial cervical spinal cord and most commonly results in pain and tetraparesis [56]. Tetraplegia and death secondary to respiratory arrest can occur [54].

The diagnosis of dens malformation may be made by plain radiographs. Oblique views may be helpful in distinguishing the dens. Myelography identifies compression of the spinal cord. Gentle flexion and extension can identify dynamic instability. A CT scan may also be used to identify malformation of the dens but is less helpful in identifying dynamic instability (Fig. 9). MRI has also been used to identify atlantoaxial instability [55] and may identify hyperintensity within the cord on T2-weighted imaging, consistent with spinal cord edema.

A number of surgical techniques have been described to stabilize the atlantoaxial joint. [54–56] Dorsal and ventral approaches are reported to have similar efficacy: 88.9% and 85.3%, respectively [56]. The ventral approach is typically favored because it allows curettage of the articular surface of the joint,

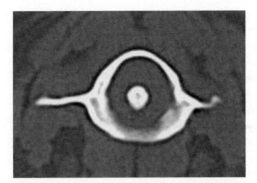

Fig. 9. CT scan of a 4-year-old Pomeranian. The dens is malpositioned dorsally, likely because of abnormal or weakened ligaments. (Courtesy of Heather Galano, DVM, Rohnert Park, CA.)

promoting bony fusion [56]. It also allows removal of a fragmented dens when necessary and may enhance anatomic alignment [54]. A small number of dogs require a second operation because of fixation failure, implant migration, or implant fracture, and this may reduce these reported success rates further. The use of polymethylmethacrylate may reduce the incidence of pin migration (Fig. 10) [54,56]. Death may occur from respiratory failure secondary to severe brain stem dysfunction after surgery [54]. Surgical failure and death typically

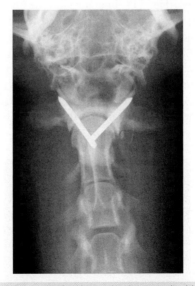

Fig. 10. Postoperative radiograph of a dog with atlantoaxial subluxation. Dens hypoplasia and/or aplasia likely contributed to instability. Threaded pins and methylmethacrylate were placed. (Courtesy of the University of California, Davis, Neurology/Neurosurgery Service, Davis, CA.)

occur within 20 days of surgery. The use of cervical braces after surgery may improve perioperative stability. Surgical success is reportedly better in dogs less than 24 months of age and when clinical signs are of a duration less than 10 months [56]. Severe preoperative neurologic signs are also associated with a worse outcome [55,56].

Intracranial Intra-Arachnoid Cysts

Intracranial arachnoid cysts have been reported in dogs and a cat [57–61]. The cysts are thought to represent an intrauterine developmental problem, resulting in splitting of the arachnoid membrane [59]. Dogs are typically less than 1 year of age at the onset of clinical signs, ranging from 8 weeks to 10 years. Small-breed dogs are most commonly affected, including the Pug, Shih Tzu, Lhasa Apso, Cavalier King Charles Spaniel, Maltese, Pomeranian, and Chihuahua [57,59,60]. Seizures are the most common clinical abnormality; however, vestibular signs may also be present [57,59,60].

MRI is considered the best imaging modality to use when evaluating for intra-arachnoid cysts [57]. CT and cranial ultrasonography through the foramen magnum, a persistent fontanelle, or a temporal window have also been diagnostic [59]. The cyst is most commonly present in the quadrigeminal cistern, an area dorsal to the midbrain, rostral to the cerebellum, and caudal to the occipital lobe. Concurrent hydrocephalus is often present [57,59]. MRI findings are consistent with a CSF-filled cyst. The cyst is hyperintense on T2-weighted imaging and hypointense on T1-weighted imaging and does not enhance with administration of contrast (Fig. 11). Imaging findings may vary if hemorrhage within the cyst occurs [58]. Two dogs presented for signs at 9 and 10 years of age exhibited intracystic hemorrhage. CSF may be mildly inflammatory, possibly secondary to prior hemorrhage [58,59].

Treatment may include medical therapy with prednisone and anticonvulsants if seizures are present. Surgical therapy is typically recommended when signs are progressive. Surgical techniques include fenestration of the cyst or shunting [57,58]. The clinical response to surgery is typically favorable;

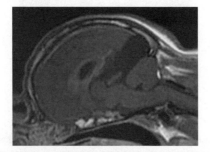

Fig. 11. Postcontrast T1-weighted sagittal image of an intra-arachnoid cyst located in the quadrigeminal cistern. Note the caudal displacement of the cerebellum.

however, results may vary. Repeat MRI after surgery may show persistence of the cyst, despite clinical improvement [58].

Spinal Malformations

Numerous congenital abnormalities that result in malformation of the spine exist. Any defect in the development and regression of the notochord, segmentation of mesoderm into somites, or vascularization and ossification of the vertebrae may lead to a vertebral anomaly. Most vertebral anomalies are incidental and do not result in neurologic signs [62].

A hemivertebra results when a part of the vertebra, usually the vertebral body, does not form. Hemivertebrae are wedge-shaped, with the base oriented ventrally, dorsally, or medially. Failure of the central portion of the vertebra to form may cause hemivertebrae on both sides, most correctly termed *butterfly vertebrae*. Hemivertebrae are seen commonly in screw-tailed breeds, such as the Bulldog, French Bulldog, Pug, and Boston Terrier. The differential diagnosis for hemivertebrae includes traumatic or pathologic fractures [63]. Hemivertebrae may lead to severe angulation of the spine, resulting in kyphosis, scoliosis, or lordosis [62].

Block vertebrae result from failure of segmentation in the developing embryo (Fig. 12). The block vertebrae are usually shorter in length than the sum of their typical individual segments. The differential diagnosis for block vertebrae includes vertebral fusion secondary to previous fracture, discospondylitis, or previous disk surgery [63].

Transitional vertebrae occur at the junction of the divisions of the vertebral column: occipitoatlantoaxial, cervicothoracic, thoracolumbar, lumbosacral, and sacrococcygeal. The defect may be unilateral or bilateral, with the vertebrae displaying the characteristics of the adjacent segment. The thirteenth thoracic vertebra may have a thick stubby transverse process instead of a normal rib. Less commonly, the first lumbar vertebra may have a rib rather than the normal transverse process. In the lumbosacral region, the first sacral segment typically takes on the appearance of a lumbar vertebra "lumbarization." The dorsal lamina separates, and a lateral process appears wing-like or similar to a transverse process of a lumbar vertebra. A new disk space is also created

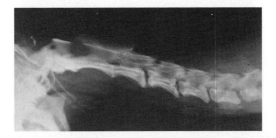

Fig. 12. Blocked vertebrae at C2 to C3. (Courtesy of Heather Galano, DVM, Rohnert Park, CA.)

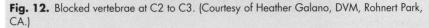

between the normally fused first and second sacral segments. The anomaly is seen at the lumbosacral junction in 2.5% to 4% of dogs [64]. In German Shepherd Dogs, the anomaly is more common, affecting 8% to 11% of asymptomatic dogs. The anomaly has been positively correlated with cauda equina syndrome in this breed. Transitional lumbosacral vertebrae have been reported in 38% to 44% of German Shepherd Dogs with cauda equine syndrome [64,65].

Diagnosis of vertebral anomalies is made via plain radiographs. When myelopathic signs are present, myelography (Fig. 13) or MRI (Fig. 14) may be used to identify secondary spinal cord compression. If spinal cord compression is present, decompressive surgery and stabilization may be of benefit when indicated. The prognosis with surgery may be guarded, because a concurrent neural malformation may be present [63] and the compression is typically chronic. In mildly affected patients, nonsteroidal anti-inflammatory therapy or an anti-inflammatory course of prednisone may be helpful.

Spinal dysraphism and congenital syringomyelia are spinal cord malformations that result from incomplete closure of the developing neural tube (Fig. 15). Clinical signs may include ataxia, a bunny-hopping gait, and decreased reflexes in the pelvic limbs [63]. Spinal dysraphism is heritable in the Weimaraner. Affected Weimaraners may have an absent central canal, incomplete separation of the ventral horns, and lack of a ventral median fissure [32].

Spina bifida is a form of spinal dysraphism in which there is a failure of fusion of the vertebral arches (Fig. 16). Spina bifida cystica, manifesta, and aperta are synonymous subclassifications in which a concurrent meningocele, myelocele, or meningomyelocele is present (Fig. 17) [66]. Spina bifida is usually incidental and is termed *spina bifida occulta* [62,63]. The condition has a relatively high incidence in the Bulldog and Manx cat and has been associated with other

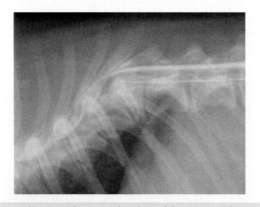

Fig. 13. Myelogram. The triangular or wedge-shaped thoracic vertebrae represent hemivertebrae. The myelographic contrast columns are attenuated and deviated dorsally at the cranial aspect of the hemivertebrae.

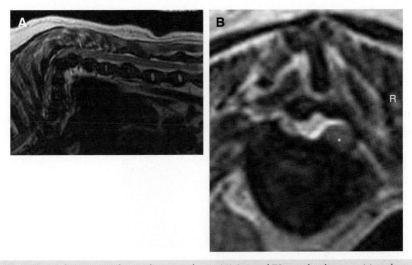

Fig. 14. Kyphosis secondary to hemivertebrae. (A) Sagittal T2-weighted image. Note the severe angulation of the thoracic spine. (B) Transverse T2-weighted image. The spinal cord (*) is displaced to the right.

concurrent vertebral malformations in these breeds. Manx cats often have sacral and spinal cord abnormalities or sacrococcygeal dysgenesis. Clinical signs of spina bifida vary based on the location of the defect. Urinary and fecal incontinence as well as paresis may be present [66]. Spina bifida cystica may be grossly evident, and in less severe cases, abnormal directions of hair growth, skin dimples at the site of malformation, or an open CSF draining tract may be present. Myelography and MRI may identify the extent of the defects. Treatment is rarely attempted [63].

Neuromuscular Diseases

The hallmark signs of neuromuscular disease are weakness, exercise intolerance, muscle atrophy, muscle fasciculations, decreased reflexes, and dysphonia. Cats with generalized neuromuscular disease often present with cervical ventroflexion. Muscular dystrophies may lead to muscle atrophy or hypertrophy and contractures. When these signs are present in a puppy or kitten, several congenital neuromuscular diseases should be considered.

Canine spinal muscular atrophy is an autosomal dominant inherited motor neuron disease in the Brittany Spaniel. Three phenotypes are recognized, causing an early accelerated (homozygotes), an intermediate (heterozygotes), and a chronic (heterozygotes) disease. Severe weakness and atrophy are seen in the accelerated form by 6 to 8 weeks of age and progress to tetraparesis by 3 months of age. Weakness, muscle atrophy, and electromyographic (EMG) abnormalities arise by 6 months to 1 year in the intermediate form. Tetraparesis ensues by 2 to 3 years of age. Clinical signs of weakness and atrophy do not

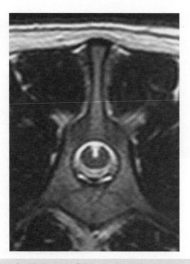

Fig. 15. T2 transverse–weighted image of the L3 spine in a 5-month-old Labrador Retriever. The dorsal funiculus is hyperintense and continuous with the central canal and the dorsal subarachnoid space, consistent with congenital syringomyelia and spinal dysraphism. A bunny-hopping pelvic limb gait and mild paraparesis were present clinically. (Courtesy of Guide Dogs for the Blind, San Rafael, CA.)

appear in the chronic form until after 1 year of age [67]. Ataxia is not a characteristic feature of the disease, because the ventral horn of the spinal cord and brain stem is affected rather than the dorsal horn, which would affect sensory nerves [68]. Muscle atrophy associated with spinal muscular atrophy is much more severe proximally than distally. Death may ensue as motor neurons in the brain stem are lost, leading to dysphagia and respiratory compromise [68,69].

EMG changes, such as positive sharp waves and fibrillation potentials, provide evidence of denervation [68,69]. Motor NCV may be normal. Muscle biopsies indicate type I myofiber loss early in the course of the disease. There is a marked variation in myofiber size, and angulated fibers consistent with denervation are seen. Motor neurons in the ventral horn undergo chromatolysis and develop internodal axonal swellings. Decreased serum vitamin E levels and increased copper serum copper levels are present in dogs with motor neuron disease. This is thought to be a result of increased oxidative stress with the disease rather than the cause [70].

Similar motor neuron diseases have been reported in other breeds. A progressive autosomal recessive neuromuscular atrophy affects English Pointer dogs. Clinical signs become evident at 4.5 to 6 months of age. Most dogs are euthanized by 1 year of age. Spinal muscular atrophy causing clinical signs before 4 weeks of age has been reported in German Shepherd Dogs and

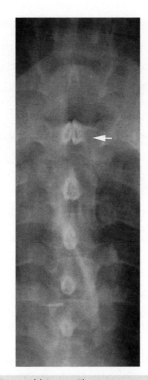

Fig. 16. Spina bifida in a 5-year-old Boxer. The spinous process (*arrow*) did not fuse at the midline. (Courtesy of Gregg Kortz, DVM, Roseville, CA.)

Rottweilers. Motor neuron diseases have also been reported in Griffon Briquet Vendeen dogs as well as in a Saluki [68].

Muscular dystrophies are a group of inherited primary myopathies and are characterized by degeneration of skeletal muscle. Muscular dystrophies may result from an absence of the muscle-associated protein called dystrophin or mutation and structurally altered dystrophin [71]. An X-linked muscular dystrophy has been described in the Golden Retriever. Variations of the disease have been reported in the Irish Terrier, Samoyed, Brittany Spaniel, Miniature Schnauzer, Rottweiler, Pembroke Welsh Corgi, German Short-Haired Pointer, Groenendaler Shepherd, and Rat Terrier as well as recently in a Labrador Retriever [72]. Puppies, generally male, are affected early and may have a stiff and stilted bunny-hopping pelvic limb gait, hypertrophic tongue, dysphagia, and trismus. Signs progress rapidly until they slow down at 6 months of age. By this time, severe weakness, atrophy, and kyphosis are likely present. Serum creatine kinase is significantly elevated, up to 100 times normal [71,73]. Muscle biopsies show nonspecific myopathic features as well as hyalinized or hypercontracted fibers, myophagocytosis, regenerating fibers, and mineralized fibers.

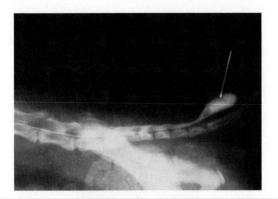

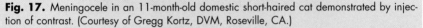

Fig. 17. Meningocele in an 11-month-old domestic short-haired cat demonstrated by injection of contrast. (Courtesy of Gregg Kortz, DVM, Roseville, CA.)

An absence of immunohistochemical staining for dystrophin and dystrophin-associated proteins confirms the diagnosis [71,72]. The disease is similar to Duchenne's muscular dystrophy in people, except for the presence of mineralized fibers [72,73].

Muscular dystrophy with laminin-α_2 deficiency has been reported in a Siamese and domestic short-haired cat. Serum creatine kinase was mild to moderately elevated in these cats [71,74]. Dystrophin-like myopathies have been reported in European short-haired cats [75]. Clinical signs of muscular dystrophy in cats are similar to those in dogs. Calcification of the tongue may be present in dystrophic cats [71].

Labrador Retriever myopathy is an autosomal recessive myopathy. The pathologic features are similar to those of other canine muscular dystrophies, with the exception of an absence in mineralized fibers. Male and female dogs are affected, and clinical signs are first seen at 3 to 4 months of age. A stiff and stilted bunny-hopping gait, generalized muscle atrophy, and carpal hyperextension are present and may progress to tetraparesis. Megaesophagus may also occur. Clinical signs stabilize between 6 and 12 months. Serum creatine kinase levels may be normal to 10 to 30 times normal [71–73]. EMG scans may show fibrillation potentials, positive sharp waves, and bizarre high-frequency discharges. Muscle biopsies indicate type II myofiber large and small grouped atrophy [73]. Avoiding cold environments and supplementation with L-carnitine at a dose of 50 mg/kg administered orally twice daily may be of some benefit [71].

Myotonia is a disorder of skeletal muscle in which there is a delay in muscle fiber relaxation in response to voluntary, mechanical, or electrical stimulation [76,77]. Puppies are affected as early as 8 to 10 weeks of age. Proximal extensor muscle involvement predominates and results in a stiff bunny-hopping gait, rigid muscles, inability to flex the stifles, sawhorse posture, and, often, marked abduction in the thoracic limbs. The proximal limb and cervical muscles are often hypertrophied. Signs may improve with mild activity and are worsened by cold temperatures. The disease has been reported in several breeds, including the Chow Chow, Miniature Schnauzer [77], Staffordshire Bull Terrier, West Highland White Terrier, Great Dane, Labrador Retriever, and crossbred Samoyed [76]. An autosomal recessive inheritance is suspected in the Chow Chow and Miniature Schnauzer [77]. Myotonia congenita has also been reported in domestic cats [25,77]. Clinical signs are similar to those in dogs [77].

In the Miniature Schnauzer, a missense mutation occurs in the gene encoding the skeletal muscle voltage-dependent chloride channel CIC-1 [77]. Myotonic muscle is hyperexcitable because of an increased resting muscle membrane resistance from low chloride conductance. Potassium subsequently accumulates in the T-tubule system, leading to excessive postexcitation depolarization and continued muscle contraction. Creatine kinase may be normal to elevated. EMG examination results in characteristic high-frequency discharges on needle insertion. The discharges repetitively increase and then decrease in amplitude and frequency, causing a sound similar to that of a dive bomber [76,77]. Muscle biopsy results vary considerably.

Treatment options include membrane-stabilizing drugs. Procainamide, quinidine, and phenytoin block sodium conduction channels [76,77]. Phenytoin also has calcium channel blocking properties [78]. Extended release procainamide at a dose of 40 to 50 mg/kg administered every 8 to 12 hours may have some benefit in reducing clinical signs in dogs [77]. Exposure to cold should be avoided. The prognosis, despite treatment, is considered guarded [76].

Storage Diseases

A number of storage diseases are caused by enzyme deficiencies that result in abnormal accumulations of various substrates. Most storage diseases are autosomal recessive disorders. With the exception of β-mannosidosis, most animals affected with storage diseases are normal at birth and gradually develop clinical signs within the first few weeks to months of life [79,80]. It is beyond the scope of this article to detail each storage disease separately. Nevertheless, it is important to keep the group in mind when a puppy or kitten is presented with diffuse central or peripheral nervous system signs with or without multisystemic disease. Tremors may be present in several storage diseases. Other organ systems may also be affected with substrate accumulations in the liver or white blood cells.

Globoid cell leukodystrophy, a deficiency of glucocerebrosidase, is seen in Cairn Terriers and West Highland White Terriers, and a similar syndrome was reported in domestic short-haired cats and a domestic long-haired cat [79,81]. The gangliosidoses are a group of lysosomal storage diseases. GM1 has been seen in Beagles, English Springer Spaniels, Portugese Water Dogs and Siamese Cats [80]. GM2 has been identified in German Short-Haired Pointer dogs and in domestic cats. Gaucher's disease, a deficiency in lysosomal glucocerebrosidase, has been reported in Australian Silky Terrier dogs.

Fucosidosis, a deficiency in α-L-fucosidase, causes enlargement of peripheral nerves in the English Springer Spaniel. α-Mannosidosis has been reported in Persian cats and a few domestic feline breeds. Several mucopolysaccharidoses have been reported. Mucopolysaccharidosis type I (MPS I) affects domestic short-haired cats and typically causes skeletal abnormalities in the pelvic limbs and a later onset of bilateral corneal opacity. MPS VI may cause vertebral abnormalities and paraparesis in Siamese cats [79].

Diagnosis of storage diseases may be based on the identification of abnormal accumulations on review of a blood smear, fine needle aspiration, or biopsy of affected organs. Confirmatory testing is also done at the University of Pennsylvania. Currently, the prognosis for storage diseases is poor. Effective treatments are not available yet; however, recent research using gene therapy shows some promise for the treatment of lysosomal storage diseases [82].

Acknowledgment

The author thanks Kris Gonzalez, DVM and Brenda Buchanan, RVT for their help with photography.

References

[1] Shores A. Neurological examination of the canine neonate. Compend Contin Educ Pract Vet 1983;5(12):1033–41.
[2] Hoskins JD. Clinical evaluation of the kitten: from birth to eight weeks of age. Compend Contin Educ Pract Vet 1990;12(9):1215–25.
[3] Beaver BV. Somatosensory development in puppies. Vet Med Small Anim Clin 1982;77: 39–41.
[4] Hart BL. Sleeping behavior. Feline Pract 1977;7:8–10.
[5] Fox MW. Conditioned reflexes and the innate behaviour of the neonate dog. J Small Anim Pract 1963;4:85–99.
[6] Fox MW. Postnatal development of the EEG in the dog—III: summary and discussion of development of canine EEG. J Small Anim Pract 1967;8:109–12.
[7] Breazile JE. Neurologic and behavioral development in the puppy. Vet Clin North Am Small Anim Pract 1978;8(1):31–45.
[8] Beaver BV. Neuromuscular development of felis catus. Lab Anim 1980;14:197–8.
[9] Kornegay JN. The nervous system. In: Hoskins JD, editor. Veterinary pediatrics dogs and cats from birth to six months. 2nd edition. Philadelphia: WB Saunders; 1995. p. 451–96.
[10] Beaver BV. Sensory development of felis catus. Lab Anim 1980;14:199–201.
[11] Jewett DL, Romano MN. Neonatal development of auditory system potentials averaged from the scalp of rat and cat. Brain Res 1972;36:101–15.
[12] Ellingson RJ, Wilcott RC. Development of evoked responses in visual and auditory cortices of kittens. J Neurophysiol 1960;23:363–75.
[13] Kovach JK, Kling A. Mechanisms of neonate sucking behaviour in the kitten. Anim Behav 1967;15:91–101.
[14] Fox MW, Inman OR, Himwich WA. The postnatal development of the spinal cord of the dog. J Comp Neurol 1967;130:233–40.
[15] Swallow JS, Griffiths IR. Age related changes in the motor nerve conduction velocity in dogs. Res Vet Sci 1977;23:29–32.
[16] Vandevelde M, Zurbriggen A. Demyelination in canine distemper virus infection: a review. Acta Neuropathol (Berl) 2005;109:56–68.
[17] Jozwik A, Frymus T. Comparison of the immunofluorescence assay with RT-PCR and nested PCR in the diagnosis of canine distemper. Vet Res Commun 2005;29:347–59.

[18] Koutinas AF, Polizopoulou ZS, Baumgaertner W, et al. Relation of clinical signs to pathological changes in 19 cases of canine distemper encephalomyelitis. J Comp Pathol 2002;126: 47–56.

[19] Moritz A, Frisk AL, Baumgartner W. The evaluation of diagnostic procedures for the detection of canine distemper virus infection. European Journal of Companion Animal Practice 2000;10(1):38–47.

[20] Inada S. Electromyographic analysis of canine distemper myoclonus. Electromyogr Clin Neurophysiol 1989;29:323–31.

[21] Saito TB, Alfieri AA, Wosiacki SR, et al. Detection of canine distemper virus by reverse transcriptase-polymerase chain reaction in the urine of dogs with clinical signs of distemper encephalitis. Res Vet Sci 2006;80:116–9.

[22] Dubey JP, Lappin MR. Toxoplasmosis and neosporosis. In: Greene CE, editor. Infectious diseases of the dog and cat. 2nd edition. Philadelphia: WB Saunders; 1998. p. 493–509.

[23] Ruehlman D, Podell M, Oglesbee M, et al. Canine neosporosis: a case report and literature review. J Am Anim Hosp Assoc 1995;31:174–83.

[24] Dubey JP, Carpenter JL. Histologically confirmed clinical toxoplasmosis in cats: 100 cases. J Am Vet Med Assoc 1993;203(1):1556–66.

[25] Dickinson PJ, LeCouteur RA. Feline neuromuscular disorders. Vet Clin North Am Small Anim Pract 2004;34:1307–59.

[26] Vollaire MR, Radecki SV, Lappin MR. Seroprevalence of toxoplasma gondii antibodies in clinically ill cats in the United States. Am J Vet Res 2005;66(5):874–7.

[27] Coates JR, O'Brien DP, Kline KL, et al. Neonatal cerebellar ataxia in coton de tulear dogs. J Vet Intern Med 2002;16:680–9.

[28] Schatzberg SJ, Haley NJ, Barr SC, et al. Polymerase chain reaction (PCR) amplification of parvoviral DNA from the brains of dogs and cats with cerebellar hypoplasia. J Vet Intern Med 2003;17:538–44.

[29] Willoughby K, Kelly DF. Hereditary cerebellar degeneration in three full sibling kittens. Vet Rec 2002;151:295–8.

[30] Kornegay JN. Cerebellar vermian hypoplasia in dogs. Vet Pathol 1986;23:374–9.

[31] De Lahunta A. Cerebrospinal fluid and hydrocephalus. In: Veterinary neuroanatomy and clinical neurology. 2nd edition. Philadelphia: WB Saunders; 1983. p. 30–52.

[32] Summers BA, Cummnings JF, De Lahunta A. Malformations of the central nervous system. In: Veterinary neuropathology. St Louis (MO): Mosby; 1995. p. 68–94.

[33] Wunschmann A, Oglesbee M. Periventricular changes associated with canine hydrocephalus. Vet Pathol 2001;38:67–73.

[34] Saito M, Olby NJ, Spaulding K, et al. Relationship among basilar artery resistance index, degree of ventriculomegaly, and clinical signs in hydrocephalic dogs. Vet Radiol Ultrasound 2003;44(6):687–94.

[35] Harrington ML, Bagley RS, Moore MP. Hydrocephalus. Vet Clin North Am Small Anim Pract 1996;26(4):843–56.

[36] Nykamp S, Scrivani P, De Lahunta A, et al. Chronic subdural hematomas and hydrocephalus in a dog. Vet Radiol Ultrasound 2001;42(6):511–4.

[37] Zabka TS, Lavely JA, Higgins RJ. Primary intra-axial leiomyosarcoma with obstructive hydrocephalus in a young dog. J Comp Pathol 2004;131:334–7.

[38] Lindvall-Axelsson M, Hedner P, Owman C. Corticosteroid action on choroids plexus: reduction in Na+K+ ATPase activity, choline transport capacity, and rate of CSF formation. Exp Brain Res 1989;77:605–10.

[39] Javaheri S, Corbett WS, Simbartl LA, et al. Different effects of omeprazole and sch 28080 on canine cerebrospinal fluid production. Brain Res 1997;754:321–4.

[40] Dewey CW. Surgical disorders of the brain. In: Proceedings of the 23rd Annual Meeting of the American College of Veterinary Internal Medicine. Lakewood (CO): American College of Veterinary Internal Medicine; 2005. p. 324–6.

[41] Kestle J, Drake J, Milner R, et al. Long term follow-up data from the shunt design trial. Pediatr Neurosurg 2000;33:230–6.

[42] Saito M, Sharp NJH, Kortz GD, et al. Magnetic resonance imaging features of lissencephaly in 2 lhasa apsos. Vet Radiol Ultrasound 2002;43(4):331–7.

[43] Zaki FA. Lissencephaly in lhasa apso dogs. J Am Vet Med Assoc 1976;169:1165–8.

[44] Greene CE, Vandevelde M, Braund K. Lissencephaly in two Lhasa Apso dogs. J Am Vet Med Assoc 1976;169(4):405–10.

[45] Rusbridge C, Knowler SP. Inheritance of occipital bone hypoplasia (Chiari type I malformation) in cavalier king charles spaniels. J Vet Intern Med 2004;18:673–8.

[46] Dewey CW, Berg JM, Barone G, et al. Treatment of caudal occipital malformation syndrome in dogs by foramen magnum decompression [abstract]. J Vet Intern Med 2005;19(3):418.

[47] Rusbridge C, MacSweeney JE, Davies JV, et al. Syringohydromyelia in cavalier king charles spaniels. J Am Anim Hosp Assoc 2000;36:34–41.

[48] Lu D, Lamb CR, Pfeiffer DU, et al. Neurological signs and results of magnetic resonance imaging in 40 cavalier king charles spaniels with Chiari type 1-like malformations. Vet Rec 2003;153:260–3.

[49] Rusbridge C, Knowler SP. Hereditary aspects of occipital bone hypoplasia and syringomyelia (Chiari type 1 malformation) in cavalier king charles spaniels. Vet Rec 2003;153: 107–12.

[50] Rusbridge C. Syringohydromyelia: pathogenesis and diagnosis. In: Proceedings of the 23rd Annual Meeting of the American College of Veterinary Internal Medicine. Lakewood (CO): American College of Veterinary Internal Medicine; 2005. p. 359–60.

[51] March PA, Abramson CJ, Smith M, et al. CSF flow abnormalities in caudal occipital malformation syndrome. J Vet Intern Med 2005;19(3):418–9.

[52] Rusbridge C. Treatment of syringomyelia. In: Proceedings of the 23rd Annual Meeting of the American College of Veterinary Internal Medicine. Lakewood (CO): American College of Veterinary Internal Medicine; 2005. p. 361–2.

[53] Vermeersch K, Van Ham L, Caemaert J, et al. Suboccipital craniectomy, dorsal laminectomy of C1, durotomy and dural graft placement as a treatment for syringohydromyelia with cerebellar tonsil herniation in cavalier king charles spaniels. Vet Surg 2004;33:355–60.

[54] Platt SR, Chambers JN, Cross A. A modified ventral fixation for surgical management atlantoaxial subluxation in 19 dogs. Vet Surg 2004;33:349–54.

[55] Knipe MF, Sturges BK, Vernau KM, et al. Atlantoaxial instability in 17 dogs. In: Proceedings of the 20th Annual Meeting of the American College of Veterinary Internal Medicine. Lakewood (CO): American College of Veterinary Internal Medicine; 2002. p. 802.

[56] Beaver DP, Ellison GW, Lewis DD, et al. Risk factors affecting the outcome of surgery for atlantoaxial subluxation in dogs: 46 cases (1978–1998). J Am Vet Med Assoc 2000;216(7): 1104–9.

[57] Vernau KM, Kortz GD, Koblik PD, et al. Magnetic resonance imaging and computed tomography characteristics of intracranial intra-arachnoid cysts in 6 dogs. Vet Radiol Ultrasound 1997;38(3):171–6.

[58] Vernau KM, LeCouteur RA, Sturges BK, et al. Intracranial intra-arachnoid cyst with intracystic hemorrhage in two dogs. Vet Radiol Ultrasound 2002;43(5):449–54.

[59] Saito M, Olby NJ, Spaulding K. Identification of arachnoid cysts in the quadrigeminal cistern using ultrasonography. Vet Radiol Ultrasound 2001;42(5):435–9.

[60] Kitagawa M, Kanayama K, Sakai T. Quadrigeminal cisterna arachnoid cyst diagnosed by MRI in five dogs. Aust Vet J 2003;81(6):340–3.

[61] Milner RJ, Engela J, Kirberger RM. Arachnoid cyst in the cerebellar pontine area of a cat—diagnosis by magnetic resonance imaging. Vet Radiol Ultrasound 1996;37:34–6.

[62] Bailey CS. An embryological approach to the clinical significance of congenital vertebral and spinal cord abnormalities. J Am Anim Hosp Assoc 1975;11:426–34.

[63] Bailey CS, Morgan JP. Congenital spinal malformations. Vet Clin North Am Small Anim Pract 1992;22(4):985–1014.

[64] Morgan JP. Transitional lumbosacral vertebral anomaly in the dog: a radiographic study. J Small Anim Pract 1999;40:167–72.

[65] Morgan JP, Bahr A, Franti CE, et al. Lumbosacral transitional vertebrae as a predisposing cause of cauda equine syndrome in German Shepherd dogs: 161 cases (1987–1990). J Am Vet Med Assoc 1993;11:1877–82.

[66] Wilson JW, Kurtz HJ, Leipold HW, et al. Spina bifida in the dog. Vet Pathol 1979;16: 165–79.

[67] Sack GH, Cork LC, Morris JM, et al. Autosomal dominant inheritance of hereditary spinal muscular atrophy. Ann Neurol 1984;15:369–73.

[68] Olby N. Motor neuron disease: inherited and acquired. Vet Clin North Am Small Anim Pract 2004;34:1403–18.

[69] Lorenz MD, Cork LC, Griffin JW, et al. Hereditary spinal muscular atrophy in Brittany spaniels: clinical manifestations. J Am Vet Med Assoc 1979;175(8):833–9.

[70] Green SL, Bouley DM, Pinter MJ, et al. Canine motor neuron disease: clinicopathological features and selected indicators of oxidative stress. J Vet Intern Med 2001;15:112–9.

[71] Shelton GD, Engvall E. Muscular dystrophies and other inherited myopathies. Vet Clin North Am Small Anim Pract 2002;32(1):103–24.

[72] Bergman RL, Inzana KD, Monroe WE, et al. Dystrophin-deficient muscular dystrophy in a Labrador retriever. J Am Anim Hosp Assoc 2002;38:255–61.

[73] Sharp NJH, Kornegay JN, Lane SB. The muscular dystrophies. Semin Vet Med Surg (Small Anim) 1989;4(2):133–40.

[74] O'Brien DP, Johnson GC, Liu L, et al. Laminin alpha (merosin) deficient muscular dystrophy in two cats. J Neurol Sci 2001;189:37–43.

[75] Vos JH, Van Der Linde-Sipman JS, Goedegeburre SA. Dystrophy like myopathy in the cat. J Comp Pathol 1986;96:335–41.

[76] Kortz G. Canine myotonia. Semin Vet Med Surg (Small Anim) 1989;4(2):141–5.

[77] Vite CH. Myotonia and disorders of altered muscle cell membrane excitability. Vet Clin North Am Small Anim Pract 2002;32(1):169–87.

[78] Grant R, Weir AI. Severe myotonia relieved by nifedipine. Ann Neurol 1986;22:395.

[79] Summers BA, Cummnings JF, De Lahunta A. Degenerative diseases of the central nervous system. In: Veterinary neuropathology. St Louis (MO): Mosby; 1995. p. 208–350.

[80] Jolly RD, Walkley SU. Lysosomal storage diseases of animals: an essay in comparative pathology. Vet Pathol 1997;34:527–48.

[81] Sigurdson CJ, Basabara RJ, Mazzaferro EM, et al. Globoid cell-like leukodystrophy in a domestic longhaired cat. Vet Pathol 2002;39:494–6.

[82] Vite CH. Gene therapy for inherited central nervous system disorders. In: Proceedings of the 23rd Annual Meeting of the American College of Veterinary Internal Medicine. Lakewood (CO): American College of Veterinary Internal Medicine; 2005.

Vet Clin Small Anim 36 (2006) 503–531

VETERINARY CLINICS
SMALL ANIMAL PRACTICE

ELSEVIER
SAUNDERS

Congenital Heart Diseases of Puppies and Kittens

Kristin A. MacDonald, DVM, PhD[a,b,*]

[a]The Animal Care Center of Sonoma, Rohnert Park, CA, USA
[b]Department of Surgical and Radiological Sciences, University of California at Davis, Davis, CA, USA

C ongenital heart disease (CHD) is a defined as a morphologic defect of the heart or associated great vessels present at birth. Abnormalities are caused by alterations or arrests in particular phases of embryonic development of the fetal heart. The term *congenital* does not imply that the defect was inherited, and the defect may have occurred spontaneously or secondary to a drug or toxin. By studying families of animals with specific CHDs, many defects have also been shown to be heritable. Additionally, if the defect was caused by a spontaneous de novo mutation, that individual has the potential to transmit the mutation to offspring. The diagnosis of CHD is important not only to the health of the patient but to eliminate affected individuals from the breeding pool.

INCIDENCE
Using the University of California, Davis, Veterinary Medical Teaching Hospital database, approximately 17% of dogs and 5% of cats examined by the cardiology service over a 10-year period were diagnosed with CHD [1]. The most common CHDs were subaortic stenosis (SAS) and patent ductus arteriosus (PDA) in dogs and tricuspid valve dysplasia (TVD) and ventricular septal defect (VSD) in cats.

CLINICAL APPROACH
The clinical approach to diagnosis of CHD follows the same fundamental principles as with acquired cardiac diseases. Signalment is important in the evaluation of CHD, because many defects have particular breed predispositions (Table 1). A history of familial cardiac disease is also important to obtain to establish a possible heritable basis of CHD. Most young animals with CHD are asymptomatic when first examined, and presence of a heart murmur is often the first clue of CHD. Syncope or exercise intolerance may be seen, and they may be ominous signs of significant cardiac disease. Cyanosis may be

*50 Windsor Court, Napa, CA 94558, USA. E-mail address: kamacdonald@ucdavis.edu

0195-5616/06/$ – see front matter
doi:10.1016/j.cvsm.2005.12.006

Table 1
Breed predisposition for congenital heart diseases

Congenital abnormality	Breed predisposition
Patent ductus arteriosus	Poodle, German Shepherd Dog, Pomeranian, Shetland Sheep Dog, Collie, Maltese, Yorkshire Terrier, Chihuahua, Bichon Friese, Keeshond, American Cocker Spaniel, Rottweiler, English Springer Spaniel
Subaortic stenosis	Newfoundland, Rottweiler, Golden Retriever, Boxer, Great Dane, German Short-haired Pointer, German Shepherd Dog
Valvular aortic stenosis	Bull Terrier
Pulmonic stenosis	English Bulldog, West Highland White Terrier, Beagle, Mastiff, Samoyed, Miniature Schnauzer, American Cocker Spaniel, Keeshond, Boxer
Tricuspid valve dysplasia	Labrador Retriever, Golden Retriever, German Shepherd Dog
Mitral valve dysplasia	Bull Terrier, Rottweiler, Golden Retriever, Newfoundland, Mastiff, German Shepherd Dog
Tetralogy of Fallot	Keeshond, English Bulldog, Wire-haired Fox Terrier
Persistent right aortic arch	German Shepherd dog, Irish Setter

identified in animals with pulmonary-to-systemic shunting defects (ie, right-to-left shunts). These animals may also have stunted growth compared with the rest of the litter. Dyspnea, tachypnea, or cough may be identified as a result of congestive heart failure.

PHYSICAL EXAMINATION

The first step to identifying a puppy or kitten with CHD is detection, localization, and characterization of a murmur (Table 2). Often, the location of a murmur and its timing may be pathognomonic for a defect or may refine the differential list of possible defects. Detection of a left basilar continuous murmur is pathognomonic for a PDA. A murmur is present in most animals with CHD, with a few exceptions, including a right-to-left shunting PDA or Eisenmenger's syndrome secondary to a large left-to-right shunt. Soft systolic murmurs (grade I–II/VI) may be heard with innocent physiologic flow murmurs because of increased flow velocity in the aorta or pulmonary artery in pediatric patients, but such murmurs usually disappear by 6 months of age. Innocent murmurs may be dynamic and vary in intensity, based on the level of activity or excitement. The murmur intensity in certain defects, such as SAS, may worsen over the first several months of life.

Other important physical examination abnormalities are alterations in femoral arterial pulses; cyanosis (generalized versus differential); signs of right heart

Table 2
Physical examination abnormalities associated with congenital heart disease

Location of murmur	Timing	Other abnormalities	Congenital heart defect
Left basilar	Systolic		Pulmonic stenosis
Left basilar	Systolic	Radiating murmur Dampened arterial pulses ± Ventricular arrhythmia	Subaortic stenosis
Left basilar	Systolic	Generalized cyanosis	Tetralogy of Fallot
Left basilar (soft)	Systolic		Atrial septal defect
Left basilar	Continuous	Hyperkinetic pulses	Patent ductus arteriosus
Left apical	Systolic	Normal pulses	Mitral valve dysplasia
		Hyperkinetic pulses	Functional mitral regurgitation secondary to patent ductus arteriosus
Left apical	Diastolic		Mitral stenosis
Right basilar	Systolic		Ventricular septal defect
Right apical	Systolic	Jugular distention/pulsation Hepatomegaly, ascites	Tricuspid valve dysplasia
Right apical	Diastolic	Jugular distention/pulsation Hepatomegaly, ascites	Tricuspid stenosis
No murmur		Caudal cyanosis	Right-to-left patent ductus arteriosus
No murmur		Generalized cyanosis	Large ventricular septal defect plus pulmonary hypertension
No murmur		Hepatomegaly, ascites Normal jugular veins	Cor triatriatum dexter

failure (ie, jugular venous distention, ascites, or hepatomegaly) and respiratory abnormalities (ie, dyspnea or increased adventitious lung sounds). Hyperkinetic bounding pulses (ie, waterhammer) are felt when there is significant aortic diastolic runoff with a PDA or severe aortic insufficiency. Conversely, dampened hypokinetic arterial pulses may be felt when there is obstruction to blood flow out of the aorta secondary to moderate to severe SAS or when there is markedly diminished cardiac output. Cyanosis occurs when the PaO_2 is 45 mm Hg or less, and this should raise the clinical suspicion of pulmonary-to-systemic shunting defects.

LABORATORY TESTS
A complete blood cell count (CBC) and chemistries are often unremarkable in animals with CHD. Animals with pulmonary-to-systemic shunting defects often have polycythemia and/or hypoxemia and may have metabolic acidosis.

THORACIC RADIOGRAPHS
Evaluation of cardiac size, great vessels, and pulmonary vasculature is useful to identify patients with moderate or severe CHD. Combined with physical

examination abnormalities, such as a murmur and femoral pulse characteristics, radiographs may be useful to narrow the differential diagnosis list. Radiographs are often normal if there is only mild CHD. Cardiac size in patients with SAS is usually normal, and thoracic radiographs may be unremarkable even in the presence of severe disease. Examination of the great vessels often reveals poststenotic vasodilation of the aorta or pulmonary artery in patients with aortic stenosis or pulmonic stenosis (PS), respectively (Figs. 1 and 2). The presence of an aortic bulge (ductal bump) near the origin of the ductus is pathognomonic for a PDA (Fig. 3). Pulmonary vascular overcirculation (ie, distention of pulmonary arteries and veins) may be detected in patients with significant systemic-to-pulmonary shunts, including a PDA, VSD, or atrial septal defect (ASD). Diminutive or undercirculated pulmonary vasculature may be seen with pulmonary-to-systemic shunts, such as tetralogy of Fallot (TOF). Animals with moderate or severe TVD often have profound right atrial enlargement and distention of the caudal vena cava (Fig. 4).

ELECTROCARDIOGRAPHY

Evidence of a normal electrocardiogram does not rule out CHD. Certain defects, such as PS or TOF, typically result in deep S waves and a right axis deviation. PDA often results in tall QRS complexes indicative of left ventricular hypertrophy. Dogs with severe SAS may have ventricular arrhythmias or ST segment abnormalities indicative of regional myocardial hypoxia. In patients with CHD causing severe atrial enlargement, there may be a supraventricular tachyarrhythmia, such as atrial fibrillation or supraventricular tachycardia.

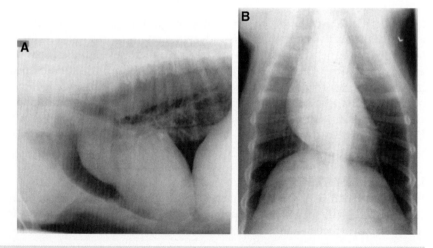

Fig. 1. Thoracic radiographs of a dog with SAS. Severe poststenotic dilation of the ascending aorta is seen on the lateral (A) and dorsoventral (B) radiographs in a dog with SAS. The heart size is normal, because there is concentric hypertrophy of the left ventricle.

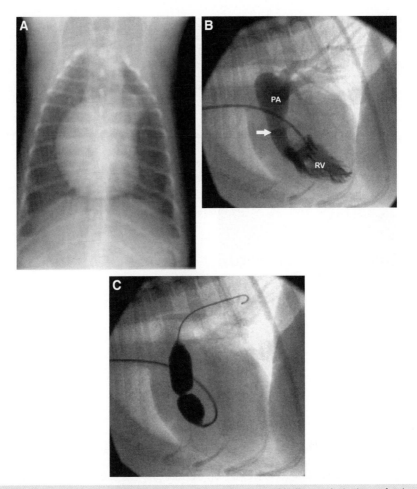

Fig. 2. Thoracic radiograph, right ventricular angiogram, and balloon valvuloplasty of a dog with severe valvular PS. (A) Right ventricular enlargement and poststenotic dilation of the pulmonary artery (1–2 o'clock position) are seen on the dorsoventral thoracic radiograph. (B) Right ventricular angiogram shows concentric right ventricular hypertrophy, a thickened and stenotic pulmonic valve (arrow), and poststenotic dilation of the pulmonary artery. (C) PS balloon valvuloplasty is performed by inflating the balloon across the pulmonic valve. The indented region of the balloon (ie, waist) is caused by the stenotic pulmonic valve, which was ripped open during balloon inflation. PA, pulmonary artery; RV, right ventricle.

ECHOCARDIOGRAPHY

Echocardiography is the cornerstone for establishing a definitive diagnosis of a specific CHD. Two-dimensional views are useful to evaluate for atrial dilation, concentric ventricular hypertrophy (ie, in response to pressure overload), or eccentric ventricular hypertrophy (ie, in response to volume overload). Careful evaluation of valvular morphology is essential for diagnosis of

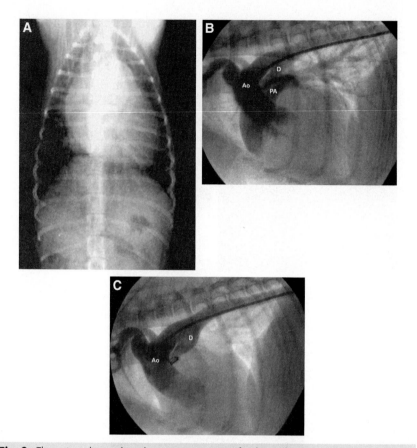

Fig. 3. Thoracic radiograph and aortic angiograms of a dog with a PDA. (*A*) Pathognomonic radiographic sign of a PDA is the ductal aneurysm (ie, ductal bulge) of the aorta on the dorsoventral radiograph. There is severe left-sided cardiomegaly and mild pulmonary overcirculation. (*B*) Aortic root angiogram shows the blood shunting from the aorta (Ao), through the ductus (D), and into the pulmonary artery (PA). (*C*) After a transarterial thrombogenic coil was placed in the ductus, another angiogram is performed, which shows a coil properly positioned within the ductus, resulting in complete ductal closure with no dye passing into the pulmonary artery.

atrioventricular valve dysplasia and valvular stenosis. Color-flow Doppler echocardiography is used to identify and localize the anatomic region of turbulent blood flow and may be followed by pulsed-wave and continuous-wave Doppler echocardiographic measurement of blood flow velocity. Noninvasive estimation of the pressure gradient between two regions is possible by measuring maximal blood flow velocity (using continuous-wave Doppler echocardiography) and is converted into pressure units by the modified Bernoulli equation:

$$\text{pressure gradient between two chambers} = 4 \times \text{velocity (m/s)}^2$$

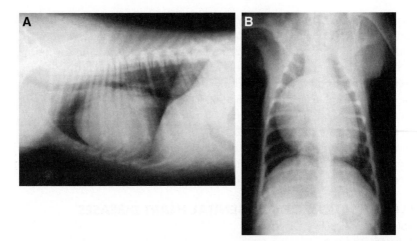

Fig. 4. Thoracic radiographs of a Labrador Retriever with severe TVD. Severe right atrial enlargement is seen on the lateral (A) and dorsoventral (B) views of thoracic radiographs. The caudal vena cava is dilated. There is increased sternal contact, increased width of the heart, and dorsal elevation of the trachea on the lateral view as a result of severe right heart enlargement. There is a loss of detail in the abdominal cavity attributable to ascites from right heart failure.

The estimation of pressure gradients is essential for determination of the severity of obstructive lesions or evaluation of pulmonary hypertension secondary to several CHDs. Positive-contrast echocardiography using agitated saline injected into a peripheral vein is a sensitive method to evaluate for the presence of right-to-left intracardiac or extracardiac shunting defects. Normally, microbubbles enter the right atrium and pass through the right ventricle and pulmonary artery to be filtered by the pulmonary capillaries. The presence of microbubbles within the left heart or aorta confirms a right-to-left shunt, and determination of the region of the right-to-left shunt is possible. For example, if microbubbles appear in the right atrium and then are seen within the left atrium, there is a right-to-left shunting ASD or patent foramen ovale.

CARDIAC CATHETERIZATION AND ANGIOGRAPHY

Given the advances in echocardiography, cardiac catheterization is rarely necessary to achieve a clinical diagnosis. Often, cardiac catheterization with pressure measurements and angiography are performed before interventional techniques for the treatment of specific CHDs, such as PS balloon valvuloplasty or percutaneous PDA arterial coil embolization. Measurement of cardiac output as well as peripheral and systemic vascular resistance and determination of the ratio of pulmonic-to-systemic blood flow (QP/QS) may be helpful to identify good candidates for surgical treatment for several left-to-right shunting CHDs (QP/QS >2.5). Surgical treatment is indicated if the main cause of the pulmonary hypertension is increased pulmonary blood flow rather than increased pulmonary vascular resistance. Right heart catheterizations are most commonly performed via a jugular venotomy or may be performed from the femoral vein. Left heart catheterizations are performed via the carotid artery or the femoral artery, depending on which interventional procedure is planned (ie, the right carotid artery is used mostly for balloon dilation of SAS, whereas the right femoral artery is most often used for percutaneous coil embolization for treatment of a PDA). Normal peak left ventricular systolic pressure and aortic systolic pressure (~100–120 mm Hg) are four times those of right ventricular pressure and pulmonary arterial systolic pressure (~20–30 mm Hg). Cardiac catheterization is useful to detect an intracardiac pressure gradient in an obstructive lesion, which correlates with the severity of the stenosis.

CLASSIFICATION OF CONGENITAL HEART DISEASES
Valvular Obstructive Diseases
Subaortic stenosis
SAS is the most common CHD of large-breed dogs (see Table 1). It is defined as an obstruction of the left ventricular outflow tract caused by a fibrous ridge or fibrotic ring just below the aortic cusps. The defect begins with small fibrous nodules of the endocardium that develop in the first few weeks to months of life, which are likely only possible to detect by pathologic examination. These early lesions are called grade 1 lesions and are rarely accompanied by a heart murmur. Over the first 6 months of life, this ridge grows and causes progressive stenosis of the left ventricular outflow tract. A grade 2 lesion is defined as a narrow fibrotic ridge that extends partially around the left ventricular outflow tract and is often accompanied by a soft grade I to II/VI left basilar systolic murmur. A grade 3 lesion is the most severe and consists of a fibrous band, ridge, fibromuscular tunnel, or fibrotic collar completely encircling the left ventricular outflow tract. There are often focal regions of myocardial necrosis and fibrosis of the subendocardium and inner half of the left ventricle secondary to the pressure overload and ischemia. There is also intramyocardial coronary arteriosclerosis, luminal narrowing, and intimal and medial smooth muscle hypertrophy in the regions of the myocardial necrosis and fibrosis [2].

SAS has been most extensively studied in a breeding colony of Newfoundlands, in which the mode of heritability was most likely autosomal dominant because of a single major gene abnormality [3]. The fibrotic defect is derived from persistent embryonic endocardial tissue within the conotruncal septum, which retains the ability to proliferate and undergo chondrogenic differentiation [2]. Mitral valve dysplasia (MVD) is the most frequent concurrent CHD.

Increased resistance to systolic ejection of blood flow through a narrowed region of the left ventricular outflow tract results in high left ventricular systolic pressure. Concentric left ventricular hypertrophy (ie, thickened walls) occurs to reduce wall stress and compensate for the pressure overload. Systolic function is usually maintained, but there may be diastolic dysfunction when there is chronic, severe, concentric hypertrophy and myocardial fibrosis. Systolic failure may be seen in aged animals with moderate to severe SAS. Myocardial ischemia may result from reduced density of capillaries within the hypertrophied myocardium, reduced left circumflex coronary artery blood flow, and systolic flow reversal of the intramyocardial coronary blood flow. The subendocardium and papillary muscles are most vulnerable to ischemia.

Exertional syncope and sudden death are common in dogs with severe SAS. Possible mechanisms of exertional syncope include activation of left ventricular pressure receptors resulting in a vagal maneuver (ie, bradycardia ± vasodilation), peripheral arterial vasodilation in the face of fixed resistance to cardiac output, or malignant ventricular tachyarrhythmia secondary to ischemia or sympathetic activation. Malignant ventricular tachyarrhythmias may occur secondary to myocardial ischemia and fibrosis and may lead to sudden death.

Dogs with SAS are likely to die suddenly within the first 3 years of life [4]. Dogs with mild SAS most often have a good prognosis with a normal life expectancy. Older dogs with less severe obstructions may develop CHF failure or aortic valve infective endocarditis. The endothelial surface of the aortic valve is disrupted by the trauma of high-velocity blood flow through the stenotic region, which predisposes dogs to develop infective endocarditis during bacteremic conditions.

The characteristic murmur of SAS is a left basilar holosystolic murmur, with an intensity that roughly correlates with the severity of obstruction. The murmur intensity may worsen over the first few months of life as the fibrotic obstruction worsens. In dogs with severe SAS, the murmur often radiates to the right thorax and carotid arteries. Femoral pulses are often hypokinetic in dogs with moderate to severe SAS because of the delay in peak left ventricular ejection. An electrocardiogram may reveal ST segment elevation or depression (>0.2 mV) indicative of regional myocardial ischemia in dogs with severe SAS. Although there is a wide overlap, ventricular arrhythmias are more common in dogs with severe obstructions. Thoracic radiographs may reveal a poststenotic dilation of the ascending aorta (see Fig. 1). Heart size is usually normal, because the hypertrophy is concentric.

Echocardiography is essential for the diagnosis of SAS and determining the severity of obstruction. Concentric left ventricular hypertrophy and a hyperechoic subendocardium may be seen on two-dimensional echocardiography in dogs with moderate to severe SAS (Fig. 5). The degree of concentric hypertrophy is poorly predictive of the degree of obstruction, however. The ratio of the cross-sectional area of the left ventricular outflow tract to the aorta has a strong inverse relation to the severity of obstruction. The right parasternal long-axis left ventricular outflow tract view is useful to identify the fibrotic narrowing just proximal to the base of the aortic valve (see Fig. 5). Color-flow Doppler echocardiography reveals turbulent systolic blood flow arising in the left ventricular outflow tract (see Fig. 5). The aortic valve is often mildly thickened, and there is always some degree of aortic insufficiency. The standard method for classification of disease severity is by measurement of peak systolic aortic blood flow velocity using continuous-wave Doppler echocardiography from the left apical five-chamber view or by the subcostal view using a Pedoff probe

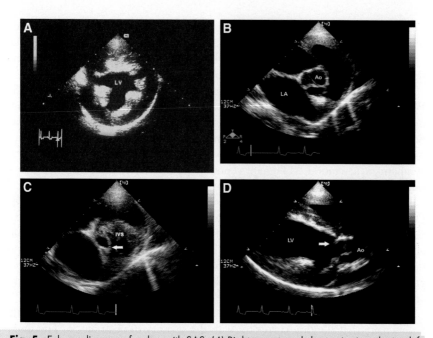

Fig. 5. Echocardiogram of a dog with SAS. (A) Right parasternal short-axis view depicts left ventricular concentric hypertrophy and regions of subendocardial hyperechogenicity consistent with myocardial fibrosis. Short-axis views depict the normal-sized aorta in cross section (B) and the severely stenotic subvalvular fibrotic ring (arrow) immediately below the aorta (C). (D) Discrete fibrotic narrowing (arrow) of the left ventricular outflow tract immediately below the aortic valve is also visualized on the right parasternal long-axis left ventricular outflow tract view. Subendocardial hyperechogenicity and concentric hypertrophy of the interventricular septum and papillary muscle are also seen. (E) Close-up view of the left ventricular outflow tract using color-flow Doppler echocardiographic interrogation shows turbulent systolic blood flow arising at the fibrotic ring in the left ventricular outflow tract. (F) Continuous-wave Doppler echocardiographic measurement of peak systolic aortic blood flow velocity (below the baseline [Ax]) reveals a high velocity of 5.5 m/s and a calculated left ventricular–to-aortic pressure gradient of 120 mm Hg, confirming the diagnosis of SAS. There is also aortic insufficiency (above the baseline [B+]), with a normal peak diastolic velocity of 4.2 m/s and an aortic-to–left ventricular diastolic pressure gradient of 70 mm Hg. Ao, aorta; IVS, interventricular septum; LA, left atrium; LV, left ventricle.

(see Fig. 5). The subcostal view yields the highest aortic blood flow velocity, but the difference compared with the left apical view is trivial [5]. Mild, moderate, and severe SAS have been defined as left ventricular outflow tract–to–aortic pressure gradients of less than 50 mm Hg, 50 to 80 mm Hg, and more than 80 mm Hg, respectively.

The most difficult aspect of diagnosis is distinguishing animals with physiologic murmurs from animals with mild SAS. In mild SAS, there may be a subtle fibrotic ridge in the left ventricular outflow tract and color-flow Doppler echocardiography may show a mild breakup in the laminar signal in that region.

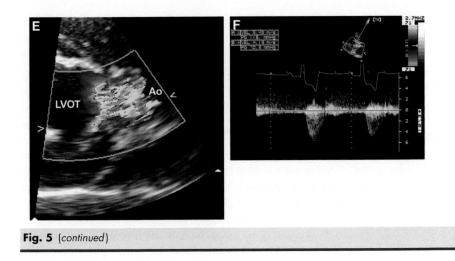

Fig. 5 (*continued*)

Although normal aortic blood flow velocity is usually 2 m/s or less, there is controversy regarding the highest limit of normal peak aortic blood flow velocity. Boxer dogs frequently have soft systolic left basilar murmurs and aortic blood flow velocities in a range of 2 to 3 m/s. Some investigators have hypothesized that these dogs have an increased sympathetic activation and increased cardiac output that lead to the increased aortic blood flow velocity in the absence of SAS [6]. Because pathologic examination to confirm the presence of mild lesions is not an option, there is an equivocal "gray zone" for the diagnosis of SAS. The presence of aortic insufficiency (in the absence of a VSD, annuloaortic ectasia, or infective endocarditis), turbulent blood flow arising in the left ventricular outflow tract with spectral broadening of the pulsed wave Doppler echocardiographic signal, and mildly elevated velocity greater than 2 m/s support a diagnosis of mild SAS.

Clinical management. Therapy is targeted to prevent sudden death and reduce syncope and exercise intolerance. The mainstay of therapy is the use of beta-blockers (atenolol, 0.5–1.5 mg/kg, administered orally twice daily) to reduce the likelihood of a fatal ventricular arrhythmia. Beta-blockers reduce myocardial oxygen demand, increase coronary perfusion secondary to the negative inotropic and chronotropic effects, and protect the diseased myocardium against arrhythmic effects of sympathetic surges. No studies have compared the effect of beta-blockers versus no treatment on survival. Extrapolation from historical control dogs with severe SAS suggests that dogs treated with atenolol live longer (median survival time of 56 months versus 19 months) [4,7]. Surgical excision of the fibrotic ring and septal myectomy under cardiopulmonary bypass effectively reduce the systolic pressure gradient but do not alter the survival time compared with dogs treated with atenolol [8]. Likewise, balloon valvuloplasty moderately reduces the systolic pressure gradient but does not alter survival compared with treatment with atenolol [7]. Perioperative prophylactic antibiotics should be given 1 hour before surgery or dentistry and 6 hours after surgery to minimize the risk of aortic valve infective endocarditis.

Pulmonic stenosis

PS is the third most common CHD of dogs and is occasionally recognized in cats. PS is caused by a narrowing of the right ventricular outflow tract, pulmonic valve, or main pulmonary artery (subvalvular, valvular, or supravalvular, respectively). Valvular PS is the most common form and consists of variable degrees of valvular thickening, fusion of the cusps, or hypoplasia of the valve annulus. Some valves seem thickened and fused at the commissures but are mobile and doming motion is observed during systole (type 1 dysplasia), whereas others are markedly misshapen, immobile, and severely dysplastic (type 2 dysplasia). Bulldogs and Boxers are predisposed to develop valvular PS or subvalvular PS secondary to an anomalous left coronary artery (R2A type) [9]. A single large coronary artery originating from the right sinus of Valsalva gives rise to the anomalous left coronary artery and the normal right coronary artery. The left coronary artery encircles the pulmonary artery and forms a subvalvular extramural compressive ring.

TVD is a common concurrent defect. Severe right heart failure occurs when there is greater than mild TVD in the face of PS. Using the University of California, Davis, Veterinary Medical Teaching Hospital medical database, approximately 10% of dogs with PS also had a right-to-left shunting patent foramen ovale. If there is significant right-to-left shunting, animals may be hypoxemic, cyanotic, and polycythemic.

PS creates an increased resistance to right ventricular systolic ejection and an elevated right ventricular systolic pressure. Compensatory concentric hypertrophy occurs in an attempt to normalize the increased systolic wall stress. Myocardial fibrosis may occur secondary to severe pressure overload and myocardial ischemia. Right heart failure often occurs if there is concurrent TVD and is likely exacerbated by diastolic right ventricular dysfunction secondary to severe concentric hypertrophy and myocardial fibrosis. Chronic severe PS may also lead to right ventricular myocardial failure.

Dogs with mild PS have a good prognosis; in the absence of concurrent CHD, they should have a normal life expectancy. Sudden death occurred in 30% of dogs with severe valvular PS in one study [10]. During exercise, dogs with severe PS have reduced right coronary artery blood flow and inadequate myocardial perfusion, which may lead to systolic dysfunction, ventricular arrhythmias, and, possibly sudden death [11]. Approximately 35% of dogs with severe PS have clinical signs, including fatigue, syncope, ascites, or cyanosis [10].

The most prominent clinical examination finding is a left basilar holosystolic murmur. If there is concurrent tricuspid regurgitation, there may be a right apical systolic murmur. Femoral pulses are usually good. Right heart failure may be present and consists of jugular venous distention, hepatomegaly, and ascites. Typical electrocardiographic abnormalities include a right axis deviation with deep S waves of leads I, II, and III as well as the left precordial chest leads. Thoracic radiographs typically show right heart enlargement and a poststenotic dilation of the pulmonary artery (see Fig. 2).

Echocardiography shows right ventricular concentric hypertrophy in proportion to the severity of the obstruction. There may be interventricular septal flattening during systole if the right ventricular systolic pressure exceeds the left ventricular pressure. There is often right atrial enlargement, which may be severe if there is concurrent TVD. The right basilar short-axis and left cranial long-axis views are useful for examination of the pulmonic valve. The pulmonic valve is typically thickened, with fused commissural cusps, and may have variable degrees of mobility with a doming motion during systole (Fig. 6). Color-flow Doppler echocardiography shows turbulent systolic blood flow and is useful to determine the location of the obstruction (see Fig. 6). Pulmonic insufficiency of variable degrees is always present. Continuous-wave Doppler echocardiography is used to determine the severity of the obstruction, with mild, moderate, and severe stenosis defined as a right ventricular outflow tract–to–pulmonary artery pressure gradient of less than 50 mm Hg, 50 to 80 mm Hg, and greater than 80 mm Hg, respectively (see Fig. 6). Dynamic right ventricular outflow tract obstruction may be seen with infundibular hypertrophy and has a characteristic late systolic peak on continuous wave Doppler echocardiography. Careful examination of the origin and course of the left coronary artery is essential for evaluation of an R2A type anomalous left coronary artery. Measurement of the pulmonary annulus diameter by transthoracic or transesophageal echocardiography is used to determine appropriate balloon diameter if balloon valvuloplasty is planned, and an ideal balloon diameter is 1.2 to 1.4 times the pulmonary artery annulus diameter. A positive-contrast echocardiogram is performed to evaluate for right-to-left shunting defects, such as a patent foramen ovale.

Clinical management. Treatment goals are to reduce the systolic right ventricular pressure overload, which may, in turn, reduce the risk of sudden death, reduce clinical signs of syncope or exercise intolerance, reduce right-to-left shunting through a patent foramen ovale, and reduce the severity of tricuspid regurgitation. Balloon valvuloplasty is a relatively noninvasive method to treat severe valvular PS. A right heart catheterization is performed, including pressure measurements and angiography (see Fig. 2). If there is suspicion of an aberrant left coronary artery, left cardiac catheterization and an aortic root angiogram may be needed to evaluate the coronary anatomy. Balloon valvuloplasty is contraindicated in patients with an aberrant left coronary artery. With the aid of a guidewire positioned across the pulmonic valve, a balloon dilation catheter is advanced across the valve and is manually inflated to tear open the stenotic valve (see Fig. 2). Repeat pressure measurements and continuous wave Doppler echocardiographic measurement of the pulmonic blood flow velocity are used to determine the pressure reduction after the valvuloplasty (see Fig. 6). Balloon valvuloplasty is associated with a 53% reduction in the risk of sudden

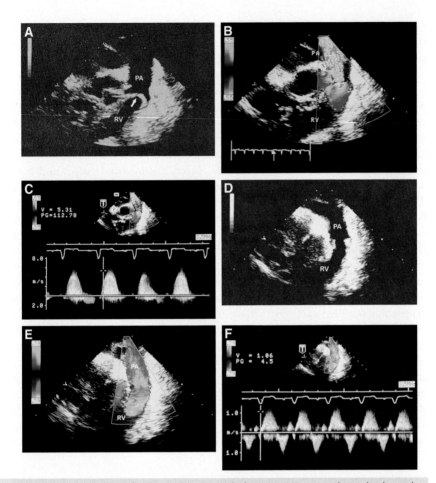

Fig. 6. Echocardiogram of a dog with severe valvular PS. (*A*) Transesophageal echocardio-gram shows the thickened pulmonic valve (*arrow*) that is fused at the commissures and domes during systole. (*B*) Color-flow Doppler echocardiography shows turbulent systolic blood flow arising at the opening of the stenotic pulmonic valve. (*C*) Continuous-wave Doppler echocar-diographic measurement of pulmonic blood flow velocity shows severe PS, with a velocity of 5.3 m/s and a right ventricular outflow tract–to–pulmonary artery pressure gradient of 113 mm Hg. After balloon valvuloplasty, the pulmonic valve is able to open during systole (*D*) and there is laminar systolic blood flow across the valve (*E*). (*F*) Continuous-wave Doppler echocardiography after balloon valvuloplasty reveals a markedly reduced right ventricular out-flow tract–to–pulmonary artery pressure gradient of 4 mm Hg and pulmonic insufficiency (blood flow velocity below the line). This is an extraordinarily optimal result of balloon valvu-loplasty. PA, pulmonary artery; RV, right ventricle.

death in dogs with severe PS and has also been associated with improved qual-ity of life [10]. Balloon valvuloplasty may be considered in less severe PS cases if there is concurrent moderate or severe TVD. Before the use of balloon valvuloplasty, surgical techniques, such as open valvulotomy under inflow occlusion or closed valvulotomy via a right ventricular approach, were used to treat valvular PS. Balloon valvuloplasty is not a viable option for the treatment of fibromuscular subvalvular PS or severely dysplastic (type 2) pulmonic valves. Surgical placement of a patch graft at the level of the right ventricular outflow tract and pulmonary artery may be the best option to relieve a muscular obstruction, but the technique confers a high risk of mortality (15%–25% with an experienced cardiac surgeon) or complications [12]. Placement of a valved conduit between the right ventricle and pulmonary artery is a possible treatment option for dogs with aberrant left coronary arteries, but there have been problems with the conduit becoming kinked within the chest cavity.

Medical treatment with beta-blockers has been advocated by some clinicians to minimize the risk of arrhythmic death. Beta-blockers also may be used to minimize a muscular dynamic component of PS after balloon valvuloplasty.

Dysplasia of the Atrioventricular Valves

Mitral valve dysplasia and tricuspid valve dysplasia

MVD and TVD are malformations of the mitral valve apparatus or tricuspid valve apparatus, including the valve leaflets, chordae tendineae, or papillary muscles, that result in valvular insufficiency. There are many types of malformations, including short thickened leaflets with clubbed tips, rolling of leaflet edges, short and thick chordae tendineae, fusion of chordae tendineae into a single chord, direct insertion of the papillary muscle to the leaflet, and upward malposition of the papillary muscle causing malalignment of the chordae tendineae [13].

MVD is most commonly seen in large-breed dogs, and Bull Terriers and Great Danes are predisposed. TVD is the most common CHD of Labrador Retrievers and has been shown to be an autosomal dominant inherited trait with incomplete penetrance, localized to chromosome 9 [14]. MVD and TVD are the most common CHDs in cats, and MVD may also be seen in conjunction with atrioventricular canal defects. Thirty-six percent of dogs and 23% of cats with TVD are concurrently affected with MVD [13].

Severe MVD and mitral regurgitation cause elevated left ventricular diastolic pressure, elevated left atrial and pulmonary venous pressures, and the development of pulmonary edema. Congestive heart failure was seen in 75% of dogs with MVD in an early study [13]. Severe TVD and tricuspid regurgitation cause elevated right ventricular end diastolic pressure, elevated right atrial pressure, and right congestive heart failure when right atrial pressure exceeds 10 to 15 mm Hg.

Clinical abnormalities and the pathophysiology of MVD and TVD closely parallel degenerative valve disease. Dogs with MVD commonly have a left apical holosystolic to pansystolic murmur whose intensity usually parallels the severity of the regurgitation. Auscultation of dogs with TVD reveals a right apical systolic murmur in dogs with moderate to severe TVD. In a study of Labrador Retrievers screened by echocardiography for TVD, however, none of the dogs with mild TVD had a murmur, making auscultation an inappropriate screening test [15]. Dogs with right heart failure may have distended jugular veins, hepatomegaly, and ascites. Electrocardiography may show various supraventricular arrhythmias, such as atrial premature complexes, supraventricular tachycardia, or atrial fibrillation. Splintered QRS complexes (Rr', RR', rR', and rr') are seen in 60% of dogs and cats with TVD [16]. Labrador Retrievers with TVD may also have an accessory pathway bridging the right atrium and the right ventricle, resulting in re-entrant supraventricular tachycardia [17]. Thoracic radiographs demonstrate variable left atrial enlargement, left-sided cardiomegaly, and, possibly, pulmonary venous distention and interstitial-to-alveolar pulmonary infiltrates of the perihilar to caudodorsal lung fields in dogs with MVD. Left-sided congestive heart failure in cats may be characterized by an atypical pattern of edema distribution or pleural effusion. Dogs with moderate to severe TVD often have profound right atrial dilation as well as a dilated caudal vena cava and hepatomegaly (see Fig. 4). Cats with TVD have right atrial enlargement and a dilated and often tortuous caudal vena cava. Cats with right heart failure may develop pleural effusion with or without ascites.

Echocardiography reveals morphologic abnormalities of the mitral valve apparatus or tricuspid valve apparatus, as described previously. There may be left atrial enlargement, eccentric left ventricular hypertrophy secondary to volume overload, and, possibly, mild myocardial failure secondary to chronic volume overload in medium- to large-breed dogs and cats with MVD. TVD may cause profound right atrial dilation that may distort the position of the other chambers, making it difficult to obtain normal standard views (Fig. 7). Color-flow Doppler echocardiography is useful to identify the presence of valvular regurgitation (see Fig. 7).

Clinical management. Medical management of congestive heart failure with furosemide (1–4 mg/kg administered orally every 24 hours to three times daily) and an angiotensin-converting enzyme (ACE) inhibitor is standard therapy. Treatment of tachyarrhythmias with antiarrhythmics may also be necessary. Intracardiac and extracardiac annuloplasty has been performed to reduce the severity of valvular insufficiency. Surgical valve repair or replacement during cardiopulmonary bypass has been successfully performed by a few highly experienced cardiac surgeons, but there is a high risk of mortality, and this procedure is limited to medium- and large-breed fully grown dogs. Dogs must remain on lifelong coumarin anticoagulant therapy [18].

Mitral stenosis and tricuspid stenosis
Stenosis of the atrioventricular valves is rarely seen in dogs and cats; if present, it occurs in conjunction with valve dysplasia and regurgitation. Atrioventricular valve stenosis is caused by narrowing of the valve orifice, which impedes atrioventricular filling and results in elevated atrial pressure. Mitral stenosis is seen in Newfoundlands and Bull Terriers. SAS is a common concurrent defect in Newfoundlands. Mitral stenosis commonly leads to left-sided congestive heart failure in almost 75% of dogs [19]. Pulmonary hypertension may occur as

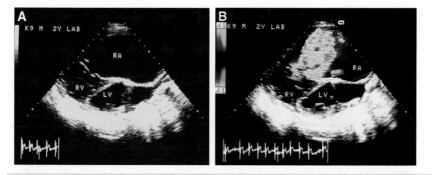

Fig. 7. Echocardiogram of a Labrador Retriever with severe TVD. (A) Severe right atrial dilation and a severely dysplastic tricuspid valve are seen on two-dimensional echocardiography. The tricuspid valve appears thickened and clubbed at the tips and is tethered by short and thickened chordae tendineae, resulting in a large gap in valvular coaptation. (B) Color-flow Doppler echocardiography of the tricuspid valve shows severe tricuspid regurgitation. LV, left ventricle; RA, right atrium; RV, right ventricle.

a result of hypoxic pulmonary arteriolar vasoconstriction and increased pulmonary venous pressure. Supravalvular mitral stenosis is a rare defect reported in cats, where a fibrotic ring or perforated membrane separates the left atrium into two chambers, with the obstructed proximal chamber usually including the auricle.

Auscultatory findings commonly include an apical systolic murmur in more than 50% of cases because of concurrent atrioventricular valvular insufficiency and, less commonly, a soft diastolic murmur in only 27% of dogs with mitral stenosis [19].

Echocardiography is necessary to diagnose mitral or tricuspid stenosis. Two-dimensional views show a restricted immobile mitral or tricuspid valve with lack of diastolic separation of the leaflets. M-mode across the mitral valve using a right parasternal short-axis view in animals with mitral stenosis reveals decreased mitral leaflet separation during diastole and a reduced E-to-F slope [19]. Color-flow Doppler echocardiography shows aliasing to turbulent mitral or tricuspid diastolic inflow and often also identifies systolic valvular insufficiency. Pulsed-wave or continuous-wave Doppler echocardiography across the affected valve shows increased peak inflow velocity and prolonged pressure half-times. The maximum atrial-to-ventricular pressure gradient is increased and may be used to quantify atrial pressure noninvasively.

The prognosis is poor for animals with significant mitral or tricuspid stenosis. In one study, 60% of dogs with mitral stenosis died by the age of 2.5 years [19]. Medical treatment consists of diuretics and ACE inhibitors, but aggressive diuresis must be avoided, because there is reliance on an increased atrial pressure for ventricular filling across the stenotic valve. Tachycardia can worsen diastolic filling and result in higher atrial pressure and reduced cardiac output, and antiarrhythmic therapy may be needed to treat tachyarrhythmias. Balloon valvuloplasty has been performed on several dogs with tricuspid stenosis, with successful reduction of pressure gradients and clinical improvement [20]. Surgical options include an open or closed commissurotomy. Supravalvular mitral stenosis may be surgically excised under inflow occlusion or during open-heart surgery under cardiopulmonary bypass.

Lesions Causing Systemic-to-Pulmonary Shunting
Patent ductus arteriosus
PDA is one of the two most common CHDs in dogs and is rare in cats. In the fetus, the ductus arteriosus connects the pulmonary circulation with the systemic circulation to bypass the nonfunctional lungs. Approximately 80% to 90% of the right ventricular output is diverted from the pulmonary artery through the ductus to the aorta. At birth, lungs inflate, the pulmonary vascular resistance drops to 20% of the systemic vascular resistance, and the blood flow reverses. Oxygenated arterial blood in the ductus inhibits prostaglandin release and triggers the circumferentially oriented smooth muscle cells of the ductus to constrict. The ductus arteriosus closes within the first 2 days of life and is securely closed after 7 to 10 days [21]. The defect responsible for a PDA is hypoplasia of the smooth muscle fibers of the ductus arteriosus [21]. PDA morphology has been divided into six grades depending on the amount of smooth muscle mass within the ductus [21]. The amount of smooth muscle cells within the ductus determines the shape of the ductus, and therefore the amount of the shunt. Nearly all ducts are funnel shaped, with the greatest amount of smooth muscle cells and constriction at the pulmonary artery end. Higher grades have less smooth muscle and less tapering at the pulmonary artery end. A grade 6 ductus almost completely lacks smooth muscle, resulting in a wide-open conduit and a reverse PDA physiology, which is discussed in the section on pulmonary-to-systemic shunting.

The amount of blood shunted across the PDA is related to the size of the ductal opening and the resistance of the pulmonary and systemic arterial beds. In left-to-right shunts, the shunt circuit includes the aorta up to the level of the ductus, ductus, pulmonary arteries, pulmonary veins, left atrium, and left ventricle. In addition to the normal cardiac output, the structures within the shunt circuit must encompass the extra shunt volume, which may be quite large in a grade 4 or 5 ductus. The result is enlargement of chambers and vessels included in the shunt circuit. If there is a large left-to-right shunt, there is elevated left ventricular end diastolic pressure, left atrial pressure, and pulmonary venous pressure, which may lead to congestive heart failure. Rarely, if there is severe volume overload of the pulmonary circulation, the pulmonary arterioles may hypertrophy and pulmonary hypertension may develop, causing the left-to-right shunt to diminish and possibly reverse to a right-to-left shunt. The window of time to repair a PDA is before development of pulmonary hypertension, because PDA closure in the face of severe pulmonary hypertension is contraindicated.

PDA is heritable in Poodles as a polygenic or threshold trait, with sex as a modifying factor (ie, female predisposition). Other breeds commonly affected are listed in Table 1. Auscultation of a PDA reveals the pathognomonic continuous murmur located in the left axillary region. If auscultation is performed too caudally at the apex, the continuous murmur may be missed and the murmur may be incorrectly classified as systolic. Femoral pulses are hyperkinetic (ie, bounding) because of the mild increase in aortic systolic pressure and the markedly reduced diastolic pressure caused by the continued diastolic shunting to the pulmonary circulation. If there is a large left-to-right shunt, the animal may be dyspneic and there may be adventitial pulmonary sounds on auscultation. Thoracic radiographs often reveal left-sided cardiomegaly and a ductal aneurysm (ie, ductal bump), which is the dilation of the aorta and the aortic region of the PDA proximal to the insertion to the pulmonary artery (see Fig. 3). An overcirculation pattern of the pulmonary vasculature may be seen. Evaluation of the lungs for evidence of congestive heart failure is essential for optimal stabilization before closure of the PDA.

Echocardiography is necessary to confirm the diagnosis, evaluate for other concurrent CHDs, and assess whether the patient is a suitable candidate for surgical or coil embolization closure of the PDA. The left ventricle appears eccentrically hypertrophied as a result of volume overload. Often, there is myocardial failure, as evidenced by an increased end systolic diameter and increased E point–to-septal separation (EPSS) of the mitral valve during early diastole. EPSS is increased with systolic myocardial failure, because there is an increased volume of blood remaining within the left ventricle at the end of systole, causing a lower left atrial–to–left ventricular pressure gradient during early diastole and reduced early diastolic flow. Less flow results in reduced mitral valve excursion and can be identified by M-mode measurement of the EPSS. Usually, fractional shortening remains normal. Myocardial failure is more common and more severe in older animals. Left atrial enlargement is generally mild to moderate. Visualization of the ductus is possible by obtaining the right parasternal short-axis basilar view and, preferably, the left cranial parasternal long-axis view of the pulmonary artery. Measurements of the minimal ductal opening size at the insertion to the pulmonary artery and maximal ductal diameter can be made by transthoracic or transesophageal echocardiography to assess whether the dog is a good candidate for coil embolization (Fig. 8). Color-flow Doppler echocardiography at the level of the pulmonary artery and ductus shows continuous turbulent blood flow shunting into the pulmonary artery from the ductus as well as laminar ductal flow (see Fig. 8). Continuous-wave Doppler echocardiography is aligned parallel to the turbulent pulmonary arterial blood flow to measure peak systolic velocity and calculate the aortic-to-pulmonary artery pressure gradient. This is useful to evaluate for pulmonary hypertension, which would result in a lower pressure gradient than expected in a normotensive animal (ie, <4.5 m/s). Centrally arising functional mitral regurgitation is often seen on color-flow Doppler echocardiography and occurs secondary to left ventricular eccentric hypertrophy and mitral annular dilation.

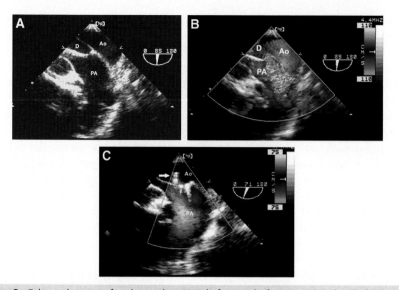

Fig. 8. Echocardiogram of a dog with a PDA before and after arterial coil embolization. (A) Transesophageal echocardiography shows the aorta (Ao), PDA (D), and pulmonary artery (PA). The ductus has a tapered funnel shape that is narrowest at the pulmonary artery end. (B) Color-flow Doppler echocardiography shows laminar aortic blood flow (*red*), laminar ductal flow (*blue*), and turbulent blood flow arising at the opening of the ductus and extending into the pulmonary artery. (C) Color-flow Doppler echocardiography after percutaneous arterial coil embolization reveals complete closure of the ductus, with no blood flow extending from the ductus to the pulmonary artery and laminar systolic pulmonary artery blood flow (*red*). The coil (*arrow*) is positioned appropriately in the narrow end of the ductus near the opening to the pulmonary artery.

Peak aortic systolic blood flow velocity is often mildly increased (ie, 1.8–2.5 m/s) because of the increased left ventricular stroke volume.

Clinical management. Treatment of congestive heart failure with diuretics is essential before surgery or coil embolization. Correction of a PDA should be performed as soon as reasonably possible to avoid the development of congestive heart failure or pulmonary hypertension. In the past, the only option to close a PDA was surgical ligation. In the hands of an experienced surgeon who has performed more than 25 PDA ligations, the complication rate is low, at less than 5% [21]. There may be silent residual flow detected by color-flow Doppler echocardiography through the ductus after the ligation procedure in 20% of dogs. Less than 2% of dogs develop recanalization that requires repeat ligation, however. Echocardiography after ductal closure typically shows a reduced left ventricular diastolic diameter, unchanged end systolic diameter, and moderately decreased fractional shortening of 18% to 25%. The left atrium is smaller and often normal in size. The ductal aneurysm usually persists, and there may be some degree of left-sided cardiomegaly on thoracic radiographs. The prognosis after ductal ligation is good. The prognosis without ductal closure is grave, and in one study, 64% of puppies died before 1 year of age [22]. Surgical closure is the only option for cats with left-to-right shunting PDAs.

Percutaneous transarterial coil embolization has become an attractive less invasive option for closure of small to moderately sized PDAs in dogs. The femoral artery is catheterized, and an aortic root angiogram is performed to identify the PDA (see Fig. 3). Under fluoroscopic guidance, a thrombogenic stainless-steel coil with Dacron fibers is positioned within the ductus at the narrowed region near the insertion to the pulmonary artery. Several coils are often placed to achieve adequate closure of the ductus. Angiography and transesophageal echocardiography are used to evaluate the amount of closure of the PDA (see Figs. 3 and 8). In extremely small animals with moderate shunts, the carotid approach may be used for coil embolization. Of the last 125 cases of attempted coil embolization at the University of California, Davis, 86% of cases had successful coil implantation, with a low mortality rate of 2.4% [23]. Aberrant coil embolization of a single coil to the pulmonary artery is tolerated without abnormalities in ventilation perfusion scans [24]. Retrieval of coils that are aberrantly embolized to the aorta or femoral artery is recommended. A considerable number of dogs may have hemodynamically insignificant residual ductal flow seen on echocardiography after coil embolization, which often reduces over the following months [23].

Ventricular septal defect

A VSD is an uncommon CHD in dogs and is one of the most common CHDs in cats [25]. VSDs can occur in several regions of the heart, most commonly in the basilar perimembranous region just below the right coronary and noncoronary aortic cusps on the left side and below the septal leaflet of the tricuspid valve on the right. Muscular VSDs are uncommon. Because the defect usually lies just beneath the aortic valve, there may be a lack of support of the aortic valve, resulting in mild dextroposition of the aorta and aortic insufficiency. Shunting across the defect depends on the size of the communication as well as the pulmonary and systemic vascular resistances. Small defects are resistive to flow, resulting in predominantly systolic shunting of flow from the left ventricle to the right ventricle. The added shunt volume is immediately ejected out to the pulmonary artery, avoiding volume overload of the right heart. The chambers and vasculature that are affected by the increased blood volume include the left ventricle, pulmonary artery, pulmonary veins, and left atrium. Congestive heart failure occurs if there is a moderate to severe left-to-right shunt. A large VSD with nonresistive left-to-right flow may lead to the development of Eisenmenger's syndrome, which is discussed in the section on pulmonary-to-systemic shunting defects.

Conotruncal malformations, including VSD and TOF, have been found to be recessively inherited in Keeshonds. In English Springer Spaniels, the heritability is autosomal dominant with incomplete penetrance or attributable to a polygenic mechanism. The cause of a VSD is unknown but likely involves lack of fusion of the muscular septum with the endocardial cushions or malformation of the conal septum. The typical auscultation finding is a loud holosystolic right basilar murmur. The murmur is not continuous, because there is only systolic shunting. The murmur intensity in an animal with a large VSD and some degree of pulmonary hypertension is softer, because there is a lower pressure gradient and velocity of shunted blood. Femoral pulses are normal. Thoracic radiographs may be normal if the VSD is small. If there is a moderate to large shunt, there may be pulmonary overcirculation and left atrial and ventricular enlargement.

Echocardiography is useful to confirm the diagnosis and to assess the severity of the shunt. In a small shunt, heart size is normal and careful inspection of the left ventricular outflow tract in the region of the membranous septum may reveal a small defect. Often, small defects are difficult to visualize on two-dimensional echocardiography, and color-flow Doppler echocardiographic interrogation of the basilar interventricular septum, including the right ventricular side, is needed to identify the turbulent systolic blood flow shunting from left to right. Continuous-wave Doppler echocardiography is used to measure the velocity of the shunt and to calculate the left ventricular–to–right ventricular pressure gradient. Knowing that the peak left ventricular systolic pressure is approximately 120 mm Hg and the peak right ventricular systolic pressure is approximately 20 mm Hg in a normal animal, the pressure gradient is 100 mm Hg. The peak systolic velocity should be greater than 4.5 m/s (pressure gradient of 80 mm Hg) in a small to moderate left-to-right VSD. Pulmonary hypertension is present if the peak VSD velocity is less than 4.5 m/s in a normotensive animal.

Atrial septal defect
ASDs are rare in dogs and uncommon in cats. Embryologic formation of the atrial septum occurs by growth of two atrial membranes. The primum septum grows from the roof the atria to the floor of the atria. The secundum septum grows from the roof of the atria on the right side of the primum septum. A defect in the development of the primum atrial septum results in an ostium low in the atria, below the foramen ovale, near the atrioventricular valves. Ostium primum ASDs are most commonly seen in cats. Atrioventricular canal defects are endocardial cushion defects that include an ostium primum ASD and a VSD. Abnormal development of the septum secundum results in an ostium at or above the level of the foramen ovale. Ostium secundum ASDs are most commonly seen in dogs.

Physical examination in animals with moderate ASDs reveals a grade II to III/VI left basilar holosystolic murmur that is created as a result of functional PS from the large right ventricular stroke volume. A split S2 heart sound may be present. Thoracic radiographs reveal right- and left-sided cardiomegaly, pulmonary overcirculation, and, possibly, pulmonary edema in large shunts. Echocardiography is necessary to determine the diagnosis and severity of the left-to-right shunt. The right atrium and right ventricle are dilated, often to a greater degree than the left atrium and left ventricle. An ASD must be visualized with the ultrasound beam perpendicular to the interatrial septum (ie, the right parasternal long-axis view); otherwise, an erroneous diagnosis might be made based on an artifact of septal fallout. Color-flow Doppler echocardiography is necessary to visualize left-to-right shunting blood across the defect, and pulsed-wave Doppler echocardiography helps to confirm the low velocity of shunting blood. A positive contrast bubblegram can also be used to identify a negative contrast jet of anechoic blood entering the opacified right atrium. The pulmonary artery blood flow velocity is mildly increased.

Clinical management. Treatment of small septal defects is not necessary, because there is a normal lifespan with small shunts. Definitive treatment of large left-to-right shunting defects is patch closure under cardiopulmonary bypass [26]. This technique is limited to only a few surgical centers in the country and is not an option for cats or extremely small dogs. An alternative to patch closure in animals with large left-to-right shunting septal defects and congestive heart failure is pulmonary artery banding. Pulmonary artery banding is used to increase the pulmonary artery resistance and reduce the magnitude of the left-to-right shunt [26]. This procedure should not be performed in animals less than 6 months of age, because the band becomes too tight as the animal grows and results in a right-to-left shunt or right ventricular failure. The band is constricted until the pulmonary artery diameter is one third the diameter of a normal pulmonary artery. Several suggested guidelines for intraoperative evaluation of the optimal degree of banding include a 50% reduction in pulmonary artery pressure and a 50% to 100% increase in right ventricular pressure [26]. Intraoperative echocardiography may be useful for monitoring the degree and direction of the shunt and left ventricular–to–right ventricular pressure gradient of a VSD. Medical treatment consists of systemic arterial vasodilation with amlodipine or hydralazine to reduce the severity of the left-to-right shunt. Palliative medical therapy with diuretics and ACE inhibitors is used for treatment of congestive heart failure. Positive inotropic drugs may be needed if there is myocardial failure, often as a result of severe aortic insufficiency.

Lesions Causing Pulmonary-to-Systemic Shunting and Cyanosis
Tetralogy of Fallot
TOF is the most common CHD causing cyanosis. Components of TOF include PS, concentric right ventricular hypertrophy secondary to the pressure overload, a subaortic VSD, and an overriding dextropositioned aorta. TOF is caused by abnormal embryonic development of the conotruncal septum, resulting in varying degrees of infundibular and valvular PS, pulmonary artery hypoplasia, malalignment of the infundibular septum, and a VSD. TOF is uncommon in the dog and cat. Genetic studies have defined TOF as a simple autosomal recessive inherited trait in Keeshonds. Other common concurrent CHDs include a PDA, an ASD, and aortic arch defects. There may be other concurrent congenital defects, including tracheal hypoplasia, peritoneal

diaphragmatic defect, pectus excavatum, retinal dysplasia, and persistent pupillary membranes. The severity of the PS and the systemic vascular resistance determine the severity of right-to-left shunting. Right-to-left shunting results in arterial hypoxemia and triggers erythropoietin production by the kidneys. The PaO$_2$ is usually 35 to 40 mm Hg in cyanotic animals. Moderate polycythemia (55%–65% packed cell volume [PCV]) is beneficial, but a hyperviscosity syndrome may occur when the PCV exceeds 70%. Bronchoesophageal arteries often hypertrophy to provide blood flow to the lungs in severe cases.

Murmur severity inversely correlates with the severity of the PS. For example, if there is mild PS and a small VSD, there may be a loud right basilar holosystolic murmur caused by the VSD shunt. Conversely, if there is severe PS, a large VSD, and a hyperviscosity syndrome, a murmur may be absent. Thoracic radiographs show right ventricular enlargement and often demonstrate pulmonary vascular undercirculation. A right ventricular hypertrophy pattern is seen on the electrocardiogram. Echocardiography reveals concentric right ventricular hypertrophy, PS (often a combination of infundibular and valvular), and, often, pulmonary artery hypoplasia. Using the right parasternal long-axis left ventricular outflow tract view, the VSD is visualized in the perimembranous subaortic region and there is a dextrapositioned aorta overriding the ventricular septum. Color-flow Doppler echocardiography is used to visualize laminar right-to-left shunting flow from the right ventricle to the aorta. A positive-contrast echocardiogram is also useful to demonstrate the degree of right-to-left shunting. Continuous-wave Doppler echocardiography is used to measure the velocity of the pulmonic blood flow and to calculate the PS pressure gradient. In the presence of a large VSD, however, the pressure gradient is not especially helpful for determination of severity of the PS because it mirrors the left ventricular–to-aortic pressure gradient (usually ~100 mm Hg).

Right-to-left patent ductus arteriosus
A right-to-left PDA is a rare CHD that is a result of large nonresistive grade 6 ductal morphology with virtually no ductal smooth muscle. Because there is a large communication between the pulmonary and systemic vascular beds, the pulmonic and systemic vascular resistances and pressures equilibrate. Irreversible pulmonary arteriolar changes occur, including medial and intimal smooth muscle hypertrophy and fibrosis, obliteration of pulmonary arteries with plexiform lesions, and microvascular thrombosis. The severely increased pulmonary vascular resistance becomes fixed and is higher than the systemic vascular resistance. Unoxygenated blood flow shunts from the pulmonary artery to the descending aorta and results in differential cyanosis of the caudal half of the body. Renal hypoxia results in erythropoietin production and secondary polycythemia. Animals with a large left-to-right shunting PDA (ie, grade 5) may develop Eisenmenger's syndrome and reversal of the PDA shunt.

Animals with a right-to-left PDA do not have a murmur, because there is laminar right-to-left or bidirectional ductal flow. There may be a split S2 heart sound secondary to severe pulmonary hypertension. Thoracic radiographs reveal right heart enlargement, a ductal aneurysm of the aorta, and pulmonary vascular undercirculation. Electrocardiography shows a right ventricular hypertrophy pattern. Echocardiography shows severe right ventricular concentric hypertrophy, interventricular septal flattening, and pulmonary artery dilation. A large nontapered PDA may be visualized using the right parasternal short-axis basilar view or the left cranial parasternal long-axis view. Color-flow Doppler echocardiography shows laminar right-to-left or bidirectional shunting blood flow within the ductus. Care must be taken to avoid the incorrect classification of a normal left main pulmonary artery as a right-to-left shunting PDA in an animal with pulmonary hypertension, however. A positive-contrast echocardiogram is necessary to confirm the diagnosis of a PDA. Visualization of bubbles within the abdominal aorta in the absence of an intracardiac right-to-left shunt confirms the diagnosis.

Eisenmenger's syndrome
Eisenmenger's syndrome occurs when there is a large nonresistive defect (PDA, VSD, ASD, or atrioventricular canal defect) with an initial large left-to-right shunt that causes pulmonary arterial hypertension and ultimately results in right-to-left shunting. Initially, the pulmonic blood flow is greatly increased because of the large left-to-right shunt. Over time, the pulmonary arterioles develop irreversible pathologic changes that result in a severely elevated and fixed pulmonary vascular resistance. Blood flow then reverses to shunt from right to left, because systemic vascular resistance is lower than pulmonic vascular resistance. This results in arterial hypoxemia, cyanosis, and secondary polycythemia.

Clinical management of cyanotic heart defects
Open surgical repair of TOF under cardiopulmonary bypass is a feasible option but has rarely been done in veterinary medicine. Surgical correction of a right-to-left shunting PDA or closure of defects in patients with Eisenmenger's syndrome is contraindicated. Avoidance of systemic hypotension is essential in animals with right-to-left shunting defects so as to avoid worsened hypoxemia. Medical management is aimed at controlling the severity of polycythemia and avoidance of a hyperviscosity syndrome. The goal of medical management is aimed at maintenance of a PCV at 60% to 68%. Phlebotomy is a useful and safe technique to reduce polycythemia. The amount of blood to be removed can be calculated using the following formula:

$$\text{blood to be removed (mL)} = [\text{body weight (kg)} \times 0.08] \times 1000 \text{ mL/Kg}$$
$$\times [(\text{actual hematocrit} - \text{desired hematocrit})/\text{actual hematocrit}].$$

The amount of blood removed is simultaneously replaced with one to two times the volume of intravenous fluids. Another alternative is removal of 10% of the blood volume in the morning without fluid replacement and removal of 2% to 10% of the blood volume in the afternoon. If phlebotomies are poorly tolerated or must be performed too frequently, reversible bone marrow suppression of red blood cell production using hydroxyurea is another treatment option. The initial loading dose of 30 mg/kg/d is given for 1 week, followed by a maintenance dose of 15 mg/kg/d. A CBC and platelet count must be performed initially every 1 to 2 weeks. Side effects of the medication include vomiting, diarrhea, anorexia, bone marrow hypoplasia, and toenail soughing. Survival is variable in animals with cyanotic heart disease and often ranges from 1 to 5 years.

OTHER CONGENITAL HEART DISEASES
Cor Triatriatum
Cor triatriatum dexter is a rare CHD caused by persistence of the right sinus venosus valve and results in a persistent membrane that partitions the right atrium into a cranial (normal) chamber and an obstructed caudal chamber. The caudal vena cava drains into the caudal obstructed chamber, and the cranial vena cava and azygous vein drain into the normal cranial chamber of the right atrium. This results in severe ascites, hepatomegaly, and hepatic venous distention in the absence of jugular venous distention or pleural effusion. This defect has only been described in dogs, and there is no breed predisposition. The only successful treatment of cor triatriatum dexter is to reduce the obstruction of the membrane manually by surgical excision under inflow occlusion or, possibly, by percutaneous balloon dilation. Cor triatriatum sinister is caused by lack of normal regression of the fetal pulmonary veins to form the roof of the left atrium and results in an obstructive membrane dividing the left atrium into a caudodorsal obstructed chamber and a cranial nonobstructed chamber. The left auricle is located within the nonobstructed chamber. This aids in distinguishing cor triatriatum sinister from supravalvular mitral stenosis. Cor triatriatum sinister has been described in cats and people. Obstruction of pulmonary venous return into the left atrium results in severe left-sided congestive heart failure. Surgical excision of the obstructive membrane under inflow occlusion or during cardiopulmonary bypass is necessary to relieve the obstruction.

Vascular Ring Anomalies
A persistent right aortic arch (PRAA) is the most common vascular ring anomaly and is commonly seen in German Shepherd Dogs and Irish Setters. Normally, the right fourth aortic arch transforms in utero to form the brachiocephalic trunk and right subclavian artery, and the left fourth aortic arch remains as the adult aortic arch. In animals with PRAA, the right aortic arch is connected to the (left) pulmonary artery by the left-sided PDA, which courses over the esophagus and trachea. After birth, the PDA closes and becomes the ligamentum arteriosum, which compresses the esophagus or trachea. A PRAA does not result in cardiovascular abnormalities. Fifty percent of dogs with a PRAA also have a persistent left cranial vena cava. A PRAA

often becomes clinically evident in weanlings that are transitioning to a solid food diet. Other vascular ring abnormalities are rare (<5%) and include a double aortic arch, retroesophageal left subclavian artery with a right-sided ligamentum arteriosum, or left aortic arch with a right-sided ligamentum arteriosum. Moderate or marked focal leftward curvature of the trachea near the cranial border of the heart in dorsoventral or ventrodorsal radiographs is a consistent abnormality in animals with vascular ring abnormalities and is not seen in animals with generalized megaesophagus [27]. Barium esophagrams may also be useful to distinguish vascular ring abnormalities from generalized megaesophagus, but misdiagnosis may occur if there is inadequate distal esophageal filling. Treatment of a PRAA is surgical excision of the ligamentum arteriosus and division of a retroesophageal subclavian artery if present. Early surgical treatment is recommended to avoid irreversible damage to the esophagus. The prognosis with early surgical treatment is fair, and dietary management is also needed.

Peritoneal Pericardial Diaphragmatic Hernia

A peritoneal pericardial diaphragmatic hernia (PPDH) is the most common congenital pericardial defect in dogs and cats. A PPDA is caused by a defect in the ventral diaphragm and pericardium that allows contents of the abdominal cavity to enter the pericardial cavity. Liver lobes and the omentum are the most common herniated structures, although the intestines, stomach, or spleen may also become herniated. A PPDH is more common in cats than in dogs, and Persians and Himalayans are predisposed. Most animals are asymptomatic, and the diagnosis is often made incidentally by identification of severe cardiomegaly with differential intrapericardial opacities, possibly including gas-filled bowel loops. In symptomatic animals, the most common clinical signs are tachypnea, dyspnea, vomiting, and anorexia. Concurrent sternal malformations, such as a pectus excavatum, an incomplete xiphoid, and fused sternebrae, are relatively common in dogs and uncommon in cats. Surgical repair is indicated in symptomatic animals.

SUMMARY OF CONGENITAL HEART DISEASES

Congenital heart defects are divided into the following main categories:

> Defects causing pressure overload
>   SAS and PS
> Defects causing volume overload
>   MVD and TVD
> Systemic-to-pulmonary shunts
>   PDA, ASD, and VSD
> Defects causing cyanosis from pulmonary-to-systemic shunts
>   TOF, right-to-left PDA, and Eisenmenger's syndrome

The clinical diagnostic workup of CHD includes proper localization and characterization of the murmur, thoracic radiographs, and electrocardiography, and a definitive diagnosis requires echocardiography. PDA and valvular PS are CHDs that may be treated successfully by surgical or interventional catheter-based procedures. Furosemide and ACE inhibitors are used for palliative treatment of congestive heart failure. Medical management of patients with cyanotic CHD consists of control of polycythemia, with the hematocrit maintained between 60% and 68%.

References

[1] Kittleson M, Kienle R. Small animal cardiovascular medicine. St. Louis (MO): Mosby; 1998.

[2] Pyle RL, Patterson DF, Chacko S. The genetics and pathology of discrete subaortic stenosis in the Newfoundland dog. Am Heart J 1976;92:324–34.

[3] Pyle RL, Harpster N, Jones CL. Genes and the heart: congenital heart disease. Proc Am Acad Vet Cardiol 1991;13.

[4] Kienle RD, Thomas WP, Pion PD. The natural clinical history of canine congenital subaortic stenosis. J Vet Intern Med 1994;8:423–31.

[5] Abbott JA, MacLean HN. Comparison of Doppler-derived peak aortic velocities obtained from subcostal and apical transducer sites in healthy dogs. Vet Radiol Ultrasound 2003; 44(6):695–8.

[6] Koplitz SL, Meurs K, Baumwart R, et al. Effect of dobutamine on left ventricular outflow tract dynamics in Boxers with soft ejection murmurs. J Vet Intern Med 2005; 19(3):416.

[7] Meurs KM, Lehmkuhl LB, Bonagura JD. Survival times in dogs with severe subvalvular aortic stenosis treated with balloon valvuloplasty or atenolol. J Am Vet Med Assoc 2005;227(3): 420–4.

[8] Orton EC, Herndon GD, Boon JA, et al. Influence of open surgical correction on intermediate-term outcome in dogs with subvalvular aortic stenosis: 44 cases (1991–1998). J Am Vet Med Assoc 2000;216(3):364–7.

[9] Buchanan JW. Pulmonic stenosis caused by single coronary artery in dogs: four cases (1965–1984). J Am Vet Med Assoc 1990;196(1):115–20.

[10] Johnson MS, Martin M, Edwards D, et al. Pulmonic stenosis in dogs: balloon dilation improves clinical outcome. J Vet Intern Med 2004;18(5):656–62.

[11] Murray PA, Vatner SF. Abnormal coronary vascular response to exercise in dogs with severe right ventricular hypertrophy. J Clin Invest 1981;67(5):1314–23.

[12] Orton EC, Monnet E. Pulmonic stenosis and subvalvular aortic stenosis: surgical options. Semin Vet Med Surg (Small Anim) 1994;9:221–6.

[13] Liu SK, Tilley LP. Malformation of the canine mitral valve complex. J Am Vet Med Assoc 1975;167(6):465–71.

[14] Andelfinger G, Wright KN, Lee HS, et al. Canine tricuspid valve malformation, a model of human Ebstein anomaly, maps to dog chromosome 9. J Med Genet 2003;40(5): 320–4.

[15] Siemens LM. Tricuspid valve dysplasia in Labrador retrievers. J Vet Intern Med 2001;95.

[16] Kornreich BG, Moise NS. Right atrioventricular valve malformation in dogs and cats: an electrocardiographic survey with emphasis on splintered QRS complexes. J Vet Intern Med 1997;11(4):226–30.

[17] Wright KN, Atkins CE, Kanter R. Supraventricular tachycardia in four young dogs. J Am Vet Med Assoc 1996;208(1):75–80.

[18] Griffiths LG, Orton EC, Boon JA. Evaluation of techniques and outcomes of mitral valve repair in dogs. J Am Vet Med Assoc 2004;224(12):1941–5.

[19] Lehmkuhl LB, Ware WA, Bonagura JD. Mitral stenosis in 15 dogs. J Vet Intern Med 1994;8: 2–17.

[20] Brown WA, Thomas WP. Balloon valvuloplasty of tricuspid stenosis in a Labrador retriever. J Vet Intern Med 1995;9:419–24.

[21] Buchanan JW. Pathogenesis and surgical aspects of patent ductus arteriosus and vascular rings. In: Weirich W, Moses B, editors. Academy of Veterinary Cardiology Proceedings. St. Louis (MO): Ralston Purina Company; 1992. p. 25–32.

[22] Eyster G, Eyster JT, Cords GB, et al. Patent ductus arteriosus in the dog: characteristics of occurrence and results of surgery in one hundred consecutive cases. J Am Vet Med Assoc 1976;168(5):435–8.

[23] Campbell FE, Thomas VP, Miller SJ, et al. Immediate and late outcomes of transarterial coil occlusion of patent ductus arteriosus in dogs [abstract]. In: European College of Veterinary Internal Medicine 14th Annual Proceedings. Barcelona (Spain); 2004. p. 191.

[24] Saunders AB, Miller MW, Gordon SG, et al. Pulmonary embolization of vascular occlusion coils in dogs with patent ductus arteriosus. J Vet Intern Med 2004;18(5):663–6.

[25] Eyster GE. Atrial septal defect and ventricular septal defect. Semin Vet Med Surg (Small Anim) 1994;9(4):227–33.

[26] Eyster GE, Whipple RD, Anderson LK, et al. Pulmonary artery banding for ventricular septal defect in dogs and cats. J Am Vet Med Assoc 1977;110:434–8.

[27] Buchanan JW. Tracheal signs and associated vascular anomalies in dogs with persistent right aortic arch. J Vet Intern Med 2004;18(4):510–4.

Vet Clin Small Anim 36 (2006) 533–548

VETERINARY CLINICS
SMALL ANIMAL PRACTICE

Selected Topics in Pediatric Gastroenterology

Michael L. Magne, DVM, MS

Animal Center of Sonoma County, 6470 Redwood Drive, Rohnert Park, CA 94928, USA

DIARRHEA

The most common causes of diarrhea in puppies and kittens are infectious, endoparasitic, and dietary. True congenital intestinal diseases, such as intestinal atresia, are rarely encountered, because affected individuals die shortly after birth.

Infectious Diarrhea

Infectious agents associated with diarrhea in young dogs and cats are typically bacterial or viral. Viral infections in dogs include canine parvovirus, canine distemper, coronavirus, and rotavirus, whereas parvovirus (feline panleukopenia), coronavirus, and retroviruses (feline leukemia virus [FeLV] and feline immunodeficiency virus [FIV]) are important in young cats. Bacterial organisms responsible for neonatal diarrhea can include *Salmonella* spp, *Escherichia coli*, *Clostridium* spp, *Yersinia enterocolitica*, and *Campylobacter* spp [1,2]. Diagnosis in most patients is usually uncomplicated and is based on typical clinical signs, serology or demonstration of virus in feces, or specialized fecal cultures for certain bacterial organisms. Treatment consists of supportive care, fluid therapy, and specific antibacterial drugs.

Canine parvovirus is the most significant cause of infectious diarrhea in young dogs; canine parvovirus type 1 (CPV-1, minute virus) is usually only considered pathogenic in puppies less than 6 weeks of age, whereas the more commonly encountered CPV-2 can cause disease in dogs of any age. Pathogenesis and transmission of the two organisms are similar. Histologic changes seen in CPV-1 are similar, although less severe, than those seen in CPV-2, and CPV-1 is capable of crossing the placenta and causing early fetal death or birth defects. CPV-1 is most commonly encountered in extremely young puppies, and presenting clinical signs include diarrhea, emesis, dyspnea, constant vocalizing, and sudden death. There are no routine diagnostic tests available, although CPV-1 infection can be confirmed by fecal electron microscopy, virus neutralization, or hemagglutination inhibition. Treatment is primarily

E-mail address: accmag@accsonoma.com

0195-5616/06/$ – see front matter
doi:10.1016/j.cvsm.2005.12.001

supportive, including fluid therapy and adequate nutrition, but is often unrewarding because of rapid progression of the disease. Prophylactic vaccines are not available for CPV-1 at present [3].

CPV-2 infection is typically seen in young dogs without protective antibody titers, because of a lack of or an incomplete series of vaccinations. A window of susceptibility also occurs in puppies, in which maternal antibody falls below protective levels but vaccine-induced immunity is lacking. A breed predilection in Rottweilers, Doberman Pinschers, and Staffordshire Terriers has been reported, and male dogs may be more commonly affected [4]. Additionally, a seasonal prevalence in the summer months occurs in temperate climates. Clinical signs of CPV-2 infection include lethargy, anorexia, vomiting, bloody diarrhea, fever, and dehydration, and the clinical course is often protracted. Leukopenia characterized by decreased neutrophil and lymphocyte counts is considered a laboratory hallmark of the disease and results from viral lymphocytolysis, bone marrow precursor destruction, and peripheral neutrophil consumption. Anemia and hypoproteinemia are common as a consequence of gastrointestinal (GI) blood loss and prolonged malnutrition. Significant secondary complications of CPV-2 infection include intestinal intussusception, sepsis, and disseminated intravascular coagulation (DIC). A diagnosis of CPV-2 infection is confirmed by virus isolation, electron microscopy, fecal hemagglutination, or fecal ELISA testing. The ELISA antigen test (CITE, Idexx, Sacramento, California) performed on fecal material is the most common and practical diagnostic test in a clinical setting; negative test results can be seen early in the course of disease, and modified-live virus vaccines can cause weak positive test results from 5 to 15 days after vaccination [5]. Treatment of CPV-2 infections includes aggressive intravenous fluid therapy, parenteral nutrition, antibiotics, and antiemetics. Fluid therapy is directed toward maintenance of hydration and control of metabolic consequences, such as hypokalemia or hypoglycemia. Colloid therapy (eg, hetastarch, plasma) is indicated in cases with severe hypoproteinemia, and blood product administration may be necessary if anemia becomes sufficiently severe. Parenteral broad-spectrum antibiotic therapy is mandatory because of disruption of the GI mucosal barrier and concomitant severe neutropenia; ampicillin or a first- or second-generation cephalosporin in combination with an aminoglycoside (eg, cefazolin, amikacin) is quite effective. Recommended antiemetics include metoclopramide as a constant-rate infusion or prochlorperazine (Table 1). Both are centrally acting agents, and metoclopramide also acts as a GI prokinetic agent. With aggressive treatment, the prognosis for recovery from CPV-2 infection is considered good, and 80% to 90% of affected dogs recover. Certain breeds (eg, Rottweilers) may experience higher mortality, however. Prophylactic vaccines are available and are effective if the manufacturer's directions are followed carefully.

The role of pathogenic bacteria in acute or chronic diarrheal disease remains unclear, because organisms may be isolated with similar frequency from healthy and ill animals. Most likely, these organisms are opportunists and establish pathogenicity when some other insult has occurred to disrupt the

GI microenvironment. The incidence of infections seems to be highest in young kenneled animals or in immunocompromised patients. Clinical signs typically include watery, mucoid, or hemorrhagic diarrhea; in some cases (eg, *Salmonella*), systemic spread resulting in sepsis can occur. The diagnosis is established by specific fecal culture (eg, *Salmonella* spp, *Campylobacter* spp) or toxin assays (eg, *Clostridia* spp), whereas in some instances (eg, enteropathogenic *E coli*), there are no practical clinically available diagnostic tests. Treatment is appropriate antibiotic therapy; however, antibiotic resistance and carrier states represent significant concerns, and a decision to treat is based on the animal's clinical status rather than merely laboratory detection of a potentially pathogenic organism [1].

Endoparasitism

Clinically significant endoparasitism of young dogs and cats includes round-worms (*Toxocara canis*, *Toxocara cati*, and *Toxascaris leonina*), hookworms (*Ancylostoma caninum*, *Ancylostoma tubaeforme*, and *Uncinaria stenocephala*), tapeworms (*Dipylidium caninum*, *Echinococcus granulosus*, and *Taenia* spp), and *Strongyloides stercoralis* as well as protozoal organisms, such as coccidia (*Isospora* spp), *Cryptosporidium parvum*, and *Giardia* spp. Clinical signs are variable and range from asymptomatic to life threatening; most common clinical signs include diarrhea, weight loss, or failure to gain weight. *A caninum* can be associated with severe hemorrhagic enteritis and anemia in puppies. Diagnosis of endoparasitic infestations is most commonly made by fecal flotation, and centrifugation techniques may improve diagnostic accuracy. *S stercoralis* may be demonstrated by the Baermann flotation technique or by observation of larvae in fresh fecal smears. *Giardia* infections can be diagnosed by observation of motile trophozoites in fresh fecal smears or by detection of cysts using zinc sulfate fecal flotation; however, a more recently developed fecal ELISA test that detects *Giardia* antigen is the preferred diagnostic test.

A number of effective anthelmintics are available for the treatment of helminth infestations (see Table 1), and routine treatment of young animals is recommended, even without diagnostic confirmation. It can safely be assumed that almost all puppies, for example, have *T canis* infection because of transplacental or transmammary larval transmission [1], and some regimens suggest treatment every 2 to 4 weeks until 16 weeks of age and then every 6 months thereafter. Control of many helminth infections can be easily accomplished by monthly administration of combined anthelmintic and heartworm preventative (eg, ivermectin plus pyrantel pamoate). Treatment of *Dipylidium* infections must include adequate flea control as well as an appropriate anthelmintic, such as praziquantel. Coccidial infections are treated with sulfa-containing drugs, such as sulfadimethoxine or trimethoprim sulfa; although frequently diagnosed and treated in the clinical setting, most coccidial infections are likely self-limiting. Fenbendazole is the recommended treatment for *Giardia* infection; although metronidazole is commonly used, it is proven less effective than fenbendazole and has greater potential for side effects [6]. A *Giardia* vaccine is also

Table 1
Pharmacologics age to for pediatric patients

Generic name	Trade name	Indications	Dosage
Anthelmintics			
Fenbendazole	Panacur (Hoechst-Roussel)	Ascarids, hookworms, whipworms, *Giardia, Taenia*	50 mg/kg/d PO for 3 consecutive days
Ivermectin	Ivomec, Heartgard (Merck AgVet)	Ascarids, hookworms, whipworms, heartworm preventative	200 µg/kg PO as anthelmintic but not approved, 6 µg/kg PO monthly for heartworm preventative
Metronidazole	Flagyl (Searle, Geneva Pharmaceuticals)	Giardia, Trichomonas	15 mg/kg PO twice daily
Milbemycin oxime	Interceptor (Ciba-Geigy Animal Health)	Heartworm preventative, ascarids, hookworms, whipworms	0.5 mg/kg PO monthly
Praziquantel	Droncit (Miles)	Tapeworms	Dogs: 5 mg/kg PO, SQ, IM Cats: 11 mg 1–3 lb, 22 mg 3–11 lb, 33 mg >11 lb
Praziquantel + pyrantel pamoate	Drontal (Bayer)	Ascarids, hookworms, tapeworms	See package insert (cats)
Praziquantel + pyrantel pamoate + febantel	Drontal Plus (Bayer)	Ascarids, hookworms, whipworms, tapeworms	See package insert (dogs)
Pyrantel pamoate	Nemex, Pfizer	Ascarids, hookworms	15 mg/kg PO
Sulfadimethoxine	Albon (Hoffman-La Roche), Bactrim (Pitman-Moore)	Coccidia	55 mg/kg PO first day, then 12.5 mg/kg PO twice daily for 14–21 days
Thiabendazole	Mintezol (Merck)	Strongyloides	50–100 mg/kg PO once daily for 3–5 days
Antiemetics			
Chlorpromazine	Thorazine (SmithKline Beecham Pharmaceuticals)	Effective phenothiazine	0.5 mg/kg IM q 8 hours 0.05 mg/kg IV (dogs)
Diphenhydramine	Benadryl (Parke-Davis)	Effective antihistamine, give before travel	2–4 mg/kg PO q 8 hours 2 mg/kg IM q 8 hours

Drug	Brand (Manufacturer)	Indication/Notes	Dosage
Metoclopramide	Reglan (A.H. Robins Company)	Gastric motility disorders, esophageal reflux, give 30 minutes before meals and at bedtime	0.2–0.4 mg/kg PO, SQ q 8 hours 1–2 mg/kg q 24 hours CRI Do not exceed single doses of 1 mg/kg
Ondansetron			
Prochlorperazine	Compazine (SmithKline Beecham Pharmaceuticals)	Effective phenothiazine	0.1 mg/kg IM q 6 hours
Antimicrobials			
Amikacin	Many	Systemic infections	10–20 mg/kg IV, IM, SQ q 24 hours
Amoxicillin	Many	Combine with aminoglycoside for systemic infections	22 mg/kg PO q 12 hours
Ampicillin	Many	Combine with aminoglycoside for systemic infections	10–20 mg/kg PO q 6–8 hours 5–10 mg/kg IV, IM, SQ q 6–8 hours
Cefadroxil	Cefa-Tabs (Fort Dodge Laboratories)	Combine with aminoglycoside for systemic infections	22 mg/kg PO q 12 hours
Cefoxitin sodium	Mefoxin (Merck)	Combine with aminoglycoside for systemic infections	22 mg/kg IV, IM
Cephalexin	Keflex (Dista Products)	Combine with aminoglycoside for systemic infections	20 mg/kg PO, SQ, IV q 8 hours
Cephradine	Velosef (Bristol-Myers Squibb Company)	Combine with aminoglycoside for systemic infections	10–20 mg/kg PO q 8 hours
Chloramphenicol	Many	Salmonella, Campylobacter, Yersinia	50 mg/kg IV, IM, SQ, PO q 8 hours in dogs, q 12 hours in cats
Clindamycin	Antirobe (Pharmacia & Upjohn)	Campylobacter, Toxoplasma, Cryptosporidium	3–5 mg/kg PO, IV, IM q 12 hours
Erythromycin	Many	Can cause vomiting, anorexia	10 mg/kg PO q 8 hours
Gentamicin	Many	Systemic infections, Shigella, Yersinia, Salmonella	2 mg/kg IM, SQ q 8–12 hours
Metronidazole	Flagyl (Searle, Geneva Pharmaceuticals)	Anaerobic infections	7.5 mg/kg PO, IV q 8–12 hours

(continued on next page)

Table 1
(continued)

Generic name	Trade name	Indications	Dosage
Trimethoprim-sulfadiazine	Septra (GlaxoWellcome)	Salmonella, Yersinia	15 mg/kg PO, IM, SQ q 12 hours
Tylosin	Tylan (Elanco)	Intestinal bacterial overgrowth	20–40 mg/kg PO q 12 hours in dogs 5–10 mg/kg PO q 12 hours in cats
Gastrointestinal protectants			
Bismuth subsalicylate	Pepto Bismol (Procter and Gamble)	Nonspecific diarrhea	10–20 mg/kg q 8–12 hours
Sucralfate	Carafate (Marion Merrell Dow)	Gastrointestinal ulceration, give 60 minutes before acid blockers	100–1000 mg PO q 6–8 hours in dogs 100–200 mg PO q 6–8 hours in cats
Cimetidine	Tagamet (SmithKline Beecham Pharmaceuticals)	Gastrointestinal ulceration, inhibits hepatic microsomal enzymes, avoid in animals less than 3 months of age	5 mg/kg PO, IV, IM q 8–12 hours
Ranitidine	Zantac (Glaxo Pharmaceuticals)	Gastrointestinal ulceration, does not inhibit microsomal enzymes, avoid in animals less than 3 months of age	2–4 mg/kg PO, IV, SQ q 12 hours can be used as CRI
Famotidine	Pepcid (Merck)	Gastrointestinal ulceration, does not inhibit microsomal enzymes, avoid in animals less than 3 months of age	0.5–1.0 mg/kg PO q 12–24 hours
Omeprazole	Prilosec (Procter & Gamble)	Gastrointestinal ulceration	0.5–1.0 mg/kg PO q 24 hours

Miscellaneous		
Diphenoxylate	Lomotil (Searle & Company)	Antidiarrheal	0.06–0.1 mg/kg PO q 6–8 hours in dogs
Loperamide	Imodium (McNeil Consumer)	Antidiarrheal, narcotic	0.08 mg/kg PO q 6–8 hours in dogs
Lactulose	Cephulac, Chronulac (Marion Merrell Dow)	Laxative, hepatoencephalopathy	1 mL/4.5 kg PO q 8 hours in dogs 0.25–1.0 mL PO q 12–24 hours in cats, adjust dose to 2–3 bowel movements per day, can be used as retention enema in hepatoencephalopathy
Dioctyl sodium sulfosuccinate	Colace (Bristol-Myers Squibb)	Laxative, 50- and 100-mg capsules	50–200 mg q PO q 24 hours in dogs 50 mg PO q 24 hours in cats
Bran		Fiber source, laxative, colitis	1–2 tablespoon in 400 gm of food q 12–24 hours
Psyllium	Metamucil (Procter & Gamble)	Fiber source, laxative, colitis	1–3 teaspoon in food q 12–24 hours

Abbreviations: CRI, constant-rate infusion; IM, intramuscular; IV, intravenously; PO, orally; q, every; SQ, subcutaneously.

available, and it has been suggested that it may be effective in clearing refractory infections [7]; however, vaccination against *Giardia* failed to decrease the incidence of diarrhea associated with giardiasis in one field study (A.D. Davidson, DVM, MS, personal communication, 2001). Some endoparasites may pose significant public health concerns, including *T canis* (ie, visceral and ocular larval migrans) and *Giardia* spp, and appropriate client counseling is advised.

Diet-associated Diarrhea

Dietary causes of enterocolitis and diarrhea in young animals include dietary intolerance, dietary hypersensitivity, ingestion of spoiled foods ("garbage gut"), ingestion of foreign material, and abrupt dietary changes. Additionally, many drugs (eg, nonsteroidal anti-inflammatory drugs [NSAIDs], corticosteroids, antibiotics, anthelmintics), chemicals like cleaning agents or fertilizers, and plants or plant toxins can cause enterocolitis and associated diarrhea. Most nonspecific enterocolitises of young animals (ie, dietary indiscretions) are acute and self-limiting, although clinical signs can be fulminant and even life threatening in certain cases. The diagnosis in such cases is usually straightforward and is based on the history, typical clinical signs, and examination findings. Symptomatic treatment is warranted in most cases before extensive diagnostic procedures, and most patients with nonspecific enterocolitis show marked improvement in 24 to 48 hours with little or no treatment. General principles of treatment include removal or avoidance of the inciting cause, correction of metabolic or electrolyte disturbances, promotion of GI mucosal repair, and control of secondary complications (ie, vomiting or abdominal pain). Dietary restriction represents the primary mode of treatment, and withholding of food for 24 to 48 hours is typically recommended. In theory, withholding of food leads to more rapid restoration of mucosal integrity and return to normal function as well as decreasing diarrhea by eliminating irritant or osmotic effects of undigested nutrients. There is an opposing school of thought that espouses "feeding through the diarrhea" on the premise that continued provision of micronutrients hastens restoration of mucosal integrity; benefits of this approach may be more relevant in secretory diarrhea, which is likely uncommon in small animal patients [1]. If clinical signs abate with an appropriate period of GI rest, gradual introduction of a highly digestible, reduced-fat, low-fiber diet is done using cooked rice or cereal supplemented with low-fat cottage cheese, chicken or lean ground beef, or baby foods. Alternatively, there are many commercial or prescription diets formulated for GI disease that may be used. A normal diet may be reintroduced over several days if clinical signs have resolved.

Bismuth subsalicylate can be used empirically as a GI protectant if necessary (see Table 1), and there is evidence that salicylates may decrease intestinal hypersecretion by inhibition of prostaglandin synthesis. Salicylate-containing compounds should be used cautiously in cats.

Parenteral fluid therapy may be indicated in some patients with enterocolitis if dehydration or electrolyte or acid-base imbalances have resulted. Attention is paid to the routine guidelines of fluid therapy: correct dehydration, supply daily maintenance, and replace ongoing losses. Hypokalemia is a common finding in patients with continued vomiting and diarrhea, and supplementation should be adjusted using frequent measurement of serum potassium levels.

Adverse Food Reactions

Adverse reactions to food may represent an immunologic reaction to a dietary antigen (ie, food allergy) or a nonimmunologic reaction (ie, dietary intolerance). Clinical signs are similar for both and include vomiting, diarrhea, or abdominal discomfort, which may be immediate or delayed in onset. Dermatologic signs, such as papules, erythema, pruritus, pyoderma, military dermatitis (cats), and eosinophilic granuloma (cats), may coexist with GI signs in patients with a dietary allergy, although this concurrence has been infrequently documented [1,8].

Diagnosis of food allergy or intolerance relies on the clinical response to an exclusion diet and recurrence of clinical signs with reintroduction of the offending dietary component. Often, the diagnosis must be considered presumptive, because many other GI diseases improve with dietary manipulations, and most clients decline rechallenge of their pets with suspect diets. Additionally, histologic changes seen in GI biopsy samples do not distinguish food allergy from other chronic mucosal infiltrative diseases, such as inflammatory bowel disease (IBD). Indirect tests for food allergy have been studied and are advocated by some individuals; however, none of these are considered reliable in veterinary patients. Such indirect tests for food allergy include measurement of antigen-specific serum antibodies (eg, RAST [radioallergosorbent], ELISA), skin testing, and gastroscopic food sensitivity testing [1,9,10].

Although dietary trials are used to diagnose food allergies and intolerances, they do not distinguish between the two, nor do they necessarily eliminate from consideration other dietary-responsive GI diseases, such as lymphangiectasia or IBD. The primary principle of a dietary exclusion trial is to feed dietary components to which the patient has not been previously exposed, and this diet should represent the sole nutrition source for the period of the trial. The recommended exclusion diet should consist of a single protein and carbohydrate source. Typically, a "novel protein" combined with rice is used; diets may be homemade, although there are also a plethora of appropriate commercial exclusion diets that consist of chicken, soy, fish, venison, or duck combined with carbohydrates, such as rice, corn, tapioca, or potato. Hydrolyzed protein diets (eg, Hill's Ultra Z/D, Hill's, Topeka, Kansas; Purina HA or LA, Purina, St. Louis, Missouri) are also available, in which proteins have been hydrolyzed into components of a molecular weight purportedly too small to elicit an immune response, although there is not proof that these diets are superior to the more standard novel protein diet. The trial diet is typically fed for a period of 3 weeks [1], although it has been shown that cases of food-allergic skin disease may require up to 10 weeks for remission. Treatment consists of continuation of a diet formulated based on the response to the exclusion trial; many suitable commercial diets are available and may be preferable because they are nutritionally balanced and more convenient.

During episodes of severe enteritis, the mucosal barrier is breached, and dietary proteins gain access to the mucosal-associated immune system; in this way, patients may become sensitized and subsequently intolerant of certain dietary proteins. Accordingly, some individuals recommend the feeding of a simplified or hydrolyzed protein diet for several weeks after such illness. Alternatively, switching to a different protein-based diet several weeks after an episode of enteritis has also been advocated.

IDIOPATHIC CHRONIC DIARRHEA OF YOUNG CATS

A refractory idiopathic chronic diarrhea is seen in young cats and is characterized by watery and voluminous small bowel diarrhea. Affected cats are usually normal otherwise and maintain a good appetite and body condition. Routine diagnostics are typically unrewarding, and the disorder may result from intestinal functional immaturity, poor feeding practices, or undiagnosed infectious or endoparasitic diseases. Treatment strategies include administration of appropriate anthelmintics and dietary trials with novel protein source foods. Fiber supplementation to the diet may be helpful in some cases, and in the author's experience, some patients may improve with antibiotic therapy with metronidazole or amoxicillin. These cases can be frustrating for the client and clinician; however, in most affected cats, resolution occurs by 1 year of age [3].

MEGAESOPHAGUS

Congenital megaesophagus is characterized by generalized esophageal hypomotility, dilatation, and unsuccessful passage of ingesta from the oropharynx to the stomach. A predilection is reported in the Miniature Schnauzer, Fox Terrier, German Shepherd, Chinese Shar-Pei, Great Dane, Labrador Retriever, Newfoundland, and Irish Setter breeds [11]. Congenital megaesophagus is rare in cats but has been seen in association with dysautonomia or pyloric dysfunction; Siamese and Siamese-related breeds have a higher incidence [12]. The pathogenesis of congenital megaesophagus is enigmatic, with some studies suggesting vagal afferent innervation defects, whereas others have suggested intrinsic esophageal biomechanical dysfunction [13].

Regurgitation is the most common clinical sign seen in affected individuals and may vary in frequency from only occasional to multiple daily episodes. Regurgitation is often described as passive or effortless and may occur within minutes to hours postprandially, and regurgitated material often appears undigested and mixed with mucus or saliva. Because of the frequent regurgitation, affected individuals are often malnourished and cachectic on examination. Aspiration pneumonia is a common complication of megaesophagus and may be reflected in fever, cough, or pulmonary adventitious sounds heard during thoracic auscultation.

Routine laboratory diagnostics are typically unremarkable in animals with congenital megaesophagus, although an inflammatory leukogram is seen in some cases with aspiration pneumonia. The diagnosis is usually easily made with survey thoracic radiographic findings in concert with the typical present-ing signs, but a barium contrast study is recommended for diagnostic confirma-tion and to exclude possible other causes of megaesophagus, such as a foreign body or congenital anomaly like a persistent right aortic arch. Endoscopic ex-amination of the esophagus is not typically considered contributory, although it may certainly confirm the diagnosis; in a small percentage of cases, secondary esophagitis may be documented by endoscopy.

Therapy for congenital megaesophagus consists of nutritional management and treatment of aspiration pneumonia episodes. A high-calorie diet in small frequent feedings from an elevated or upright position is recommended. A pe-riod of trial and error may be needed to determine the most appropriate dietary consistency, because some individuals tolerate a completely liquid diet best, whereas others perform better when given solid foods. Being held in an upright position for 15 to 30 minutes after eating may be helpful in some animals by facilitating gravity drainage of the esophagus. Individuals that cannot maintain an adequate nutritional level orally may require gastrostomy tube placement, surgically or endoscopically, for feeding.

Aspiration pneumonia is treated with appropriate antibiotic therapy, which is ideally selected on the basis of culture and sensitivity of samples collected by a tracheal wash or endoscopic bronchoalveolar lavage. Supportive treatment measures for aspiration pneumonia include supplemental oxygen administra-tion, thoracic coupage, and perhaps nebulization therapy. It is recommended that antibiotic therapy be continued for at least 7 to 10 days beyond radio-graphic resolution of the pneumonia.

GI prokinetic agents, such as metoclopramide and cisapride, have been used empirically in the treatment of megaesophagus; however, they typically result in significant worsening of signs of regurgitation. This clinical worsening occurs from a marked increase in lower esophageal sphincter resting pressure in re-sponse to these drugs, thereby increasing resistance to esophageal outflow, whereas improvement in esophageal motility, if any, is insubstantial.

The prognosis for congenital megaesophagus is considered fair. Many affected animals eventually show improvement in esophageal motility and function if adequate nutritional support is provided. Repeated episodes of aspiration pneu-monia are, unfortunately, common, and a decision to euthanatize because of these is a leading cause of mortality.

PORTOSYSTEMIC SHUNTS

A portosystemic shunt (PSS) is a congenital malformation of the hepatic portal venous drainage system and can have a familial (ie, genetic) or random occur-rence. A congenital PSS can be intrahepatic or extrahepatic; breed predilections for extrahepatic shunts include the Yorkshire Terrier, Maltese, Poodle, Minia-ture Schnauzer, Dachshund, Lhasa Apso, Pekingese, Pug, and Shih Tzu. Intra-hepatic shunts are more commonly identified in large-breed dogs, such as Golden Retrievers, German Shepherds, Irish Wolfhounds, Irish Setters, and Samoyeds [14]. PSSs are uncommon in cats.

Clinical signs attributable to a PSS are most often seen before 2 years of age, although they may not be evident in some individuals until much later in life. Clinical signs of a PSS result from loss of hepatic metabolic functions and often include drug (anesthetics or sedatives) intolerance, hepatic encephalopathy, anorexia, vomiting, and diarrhea. Hepatic encephalopathy may lead to seizures, stupor, coma, amaurosis, or mentation changes. Ammonium biurate urinary calculi may develop in some individuals and can cause stranguria, pollakiuria, and hematuria, and the finding of urate calculi in a non-Dalmation breed should raise suspicion of a PSS. Individuals with a PSS are often stunted in growth. Ptyalism is often a prominent clinical sign in cats with PSSs. Other clinical findings in cats include cardiac murmurs, renomegaly, and a characteristic "golden" or copper discoloration of the iris [15].

Biochemical abnormalities commonly associated with a PSS include mild to moderate liver enzyme elevations, hypoglycemia, low blood urea nitrogen (BUN), hypoalbuminemia, and hypocholesterolemia. Red blood cell microcytosis or mild nonregenerative anemia may be seen. Ammonium biurate crystalluria, hematuria, and pyuria can occur in animals with urate uroliths. Although uncommon, routine blood work and urinalysis can be completely normal in some individuals with a PSS. Other tests of liver function include measurement of serum bile acids and blood ammonia levels. Bile acid tolerance testing is recommended, in which fasting and 2-hour postprandial levels are measured. Although not pathognomic for a PSS, marked elevations in bile acid levels are characteristic and should greatly elevate the index of suspicion in patients of appropriate age and clinical presentation. Blood ammonia levels are measured postprandially after ingestion of a high-protein meal or after oral ammonia challenge, and hyperammonemia is a frequent finding.

Abdominal ultrasonography is a useful diagnostic technique and is routinely done when a PSS is suspected. It is noninvasive and requires no anesthesia; however, diagnostic accuracy is highly operator dependent, and the PSS is confirmed in only approximately 60% to 80% of cases [16]. Transcolonic portal scintigraphy is another useful diagnostic tool and has a high degree of accuracy. Disadvantages include limited availability, extensive patient preparation, and the potential need for sedation or anesthesia during the procedure. Transsplenic portography after intrasplenic contrast material injection can also be used to identify a PSS successfully and is a relatively simple procedure, although it also does require anesthesia. Finally, mesenteric portography, although it is the most invasive technique and requires general anesthesia, is a highly reliable method of confirming and localizing a PSS.

Treatment of a PSS may be palliative by medical management or definitive by surgical ligation. It must be emphasized that medical management is only a symptomatic therapy and that a delay in surgical ligation may lead to further deterioration in liver function or ability to recover after shunt ligation.

Medical therapy of patients with a PSS is directed primarily at controlling signs of hepatoencephalopathy (HE) by limiting absorption of toxins from the GI tract and manipulation of dietary proteins. Lactulose is a nonabsorbed synthetic disaccharide that is degraded to organic acids by colonic bacteria. This leads to a decrease in colonic luminal pH, resulting in ionic trapping of ammonia as ammonium ion, which is incapable of diffusing into the portal circulation. Additionally, the organic acid byproducts of lactulose digestion act as an osmotic cathartic, thereby decreasing colon retention time and absorption of toxic metabolites. Lactulose as well as neomycin or povidone iodine may be used in retention enemas in the treatment of patients in encephalopathic crisis. Antibiotics like metronidazole, neomycin, ampicillin, or amoxicillin are routinely used to suppress intestinal anaerobic flora responsible for enteric ammonia production (see Table 1).

Blood within the GI tract is a potent source of ammonia production, and treatment of GI hemorrhage is a key component in the successful management of HE. Treatment considerations include H_2-receptor blockers or proton-pump inhibitors to decrease acid secretion, coating agents like sucralfate (see Table 1), and treatment of any primary causes like endoparasitism.

Restriction of dietary protein intake is a critical element of the medical management of a PSS. Diets high in branched-chain amino acids and limited in aromatic amino acids are recommended, with a recommended daily protein intake of 2.0 to 2.5 mg/kg [15]. Milk and vegetable proteins, such as cottage cheese and tofu, are excellent protein sources, with the bulk of dietary caloric intake consisting of carbohydrates, such as boiled white rice. Small frequent feedings are recommended to maximize digestion and absorption. Commercial low-protein diets, such as L/D, K/D or I/D (Hill's, Topeka, Kansas), are suitable for use in dogs and cats with a PSS, and there are also homemade diets that can be beneficial.

Surgical shunt ligation is the definitive treatment for a PSS, and the current recommended method of ligation is by placement of an amaroid constrictor. The amaroid constrictor consists of a dehydrated casein core surrounded by a metal ring. After placement of the amaroid constrictor, the casein core absorbs water and enlarges, leading to gradual occlusion of the shunting vessel over a period of several weeks to months. This avoids the major complication of portal hypertension seen in many cases after abrupt shunt occlusion. Postoperative complications are uncommon but can include portal hypertension, postoperative seizures, or rupture of the shunting vessel, all of which have a high mortality rate; however, overall mortality with surgical shunt ligation is less than 10%.

CHRONIC ENTEROPATHIES

A genetic predilection to small intestinal disease has been reported in several breeds of dogs. An immunoproliferative enteropathy is seen in the Basenji breed, which is characterized by lymphangiectasia, intermittent diarrhea, weight loss, hypoalbuminemia and hyperglobulinemia, and lymphoplasmacytic mucosal infiltrates throughout the GI tract [17]. Other reported clinical signs include paresis, seizures, facial muscle contracture, buccal lymphadenomegaly, and adverse vaccine reactions. The diagnosis is confirmed by intestinal histopathologic examination obtained via a laparotomy or endoscopically obtained biopsy samples. Treatment options include dietary manipulation, corticosteroids, and antibiotic therapy. Diets are typically formulated as fat restricted and high-quality protein and may include commercial GI diets, weight control diets, or appropriate homemade formulas. Frequent small feedings and fat-soluble vitamin supplementation are recommended. Medium-chain triglycerides are used as a dietary caloric source that bypasses lymphatic absorption and are usually added to the diet in an oil form; however, vomiting and diarrhea can be problematic side effects. Corticosteroids are usually administered initially at a higher dosage to "induce remission" and are then tapered slowly to a lower and more tolerable maintenance level. Antibiotic therapy with agents like metronidazole, amoxicillin, or tylosin (see Table 1) may be beneficial in individuals with suspected or confirmed bacterial overgrowth.

Wheat-sensitive or gluten enteropathy has been reported in Irish Setter dogs and is clinically typified by weight loss or poor weight gain as well as by intermittent diarrhea episodes [18,19]. This disorder is attributable to selective deficiencies in certain brush border enzymes, resulting in hypersensitivity to wheat in the diet. Histopathologic changes are often patchy or segmental and are typified by villous atrophy without a significant inflammatory infiltrate. Treatment is elimination of wheat from the diet.

Chinese Sharpei dogs have been identified with an enteropathy that is characterized by poor weight gain, weight loss, or intermittent diarrhea episodes, with onset of signs typically between 2 and 6 months of age [2]. Histopathologic examination of intestinal biopsy samples shows lymphoplasmacytic-eosinophilic mucosal infiltrates. Treatment is dietary management and immunosuppressive therapy with corticosteroids; however, the response to therapy is variable, and more potent immunosuppressives, such as azathioprine, may be necessary in certain individuals. Bacterial overgrowth is not infrequent, as reflected in elevated serum folate and decreased serum cobalamin levels, and some affected dogs may benefit from long-term antibiotic therapy.

Selective cobalamin malabsorption has been identified in Giant Schnauzer dogs with clinical signs of anorexia, lethargy, and poor weight gain or weight loss, usually beginning between 3 and 6 months of age; nonregenerative megaloblastic anemia and neutropenia are also characteristic [20]. This disorder results from a defect in transport of the intrinsic factor cobalamin receptor complex to the brush border membrane in the ileum. Treatment is parenteral cobalamin administration weekly for 4 to 6 weeks and then every 3 months thereafter. Recovery is usually complete.

JUVENILE PANCREATIC ATROPHY

Pancreatic atrophy or hypoplasia of unknown but perhaps genetic cause is reported in young dogs; German Shepherd dogs are predisposed, accounting for approximately one half of the reported cases [21]. Pancreatic exocrine insufficiency (PEI) results, and clinical signs of diarrhea, weight loss, and steatorrhea usually develop between 6 and 12 of age. Diagnosis is typically straightforward and is established by finding markedly decreased serum trypsin–like immuno-reactivity levels.

Primary treatment consists of dietary pancreatic enzyme replacement using agents like pancreatin or pancrelipase. Powdered formulations or crushed non–enteric-coated tablets are recommended, because absorption of enteric-coated tablets is unpredictable. Mixing of pancreatic enzyme replacements with food 30 to 60 minutes before feeding is recommended so as to circumvent the loss of enzyme activity that occurs in the stomach. Reduced-fat high-carbohydrate diets are typically recommended, because lipids are the most severely mal-absorbed dietary nutrient; however, some afflicted individuals respond better to non–fat-restricted diets. Frequent smaller feedings (eg, three times a day) are recommended. High-fiber diets are avoided, because dietary fiber has been shown to decrease intestinal pancreatic enzyme activity and perhaps pancreatic secretion.

Many patients also benefit from acid secretion inhibition with drugs like ci-metidine, ranitidine, famotidine, or omeprazole (see Table 1). Intestinal bacterial overgrowth often accompanies PEI, and antibiotic therapy may be useful in refractory patients. The prognosis for PEI is considered good.

References

[1] Hall EJ, German AJ. Diseases of the small intestine. In: Ettinger SJ, Feldman EC, editors. Text-book of veterinary internal medicine. 6th edition. Philadelphia: WB Saunders; 2005. p. 1332–78.

[2] Hoskins JD, Dimski D. The digestive system. In: Hoskins JD, editor. Veterinary pediatrics. 2nd edition. Philadelphia: WB Saunders; 1990. p. 133–87.

[3] Hoskins JD. Neonatal diarrhea in puppies and kittens. In: Bonagura JD, editor. Kirk's current veterinary therapy XIII. Philadelphia: WB Saunders; 2000. p. 625–8.

[4] Glickman LT, Domanski LM, Patronek GI, et al. Breed-related risk factors for canine parvo-virus enteritis. J Am Vet Med Assoc 1985;187:589–91.

[5] Rewerts JM, Cohn LA. CVT update: diagnosis and treatment of parvovirus. In: Bonagura JD, editor. Kirk's current veterinary therapy XIII. Philadelphia: WB Saunders; 2000. p. 629–32.

[6] Barr SC, Bowman DD, Heller RL. Efficiency of fenbendazole against giardiasis in dogs. Am J Vet Res 1994;55:998–9.

[7] Olson ME, Hanniogan CJ, Gaviller PF, et al. The use of a giardia vaccine as an immunother-apeutic agent in dogs. Can Vet J 2001;43:865–8.

[8] Paterson S. Food hypersensitivity in 20 dogs with skin and gastrointestinal signs. J Small Anim Pract 1995;36:529–34.

[9] Foster AP, Knowles TG, Moore AH, et al. Serum IgE responses to food antigens in normal and atopic dogs, and dogs with gastrointestinal disease. Vet Immunol Immunopathol 2003;92:123–4.

[10] Bischoff SC, Mayer J, Wedemeyer, et al. Colonoscopic allergen provocation (COLAP): a new diagnostic approach for gastrointestinal food allergy. Gut 1997;40:745–53.

[11] Strombeck DR, Guilford WG. Diseases of swallowing. In: Small animal gastroenterology. 2nd edition. Davis (CA): Stonegate Publishing; 1990. p. 140–66.

[12] Watrous BJ. Esophageal disease. In: Ettinger SJ, editor. Textbook of veterinary internal medicine. 2nd edition. Philadelphia: WB Saunders; 1983. p. 1191.

[13] Holland CT, Satchell PM, Farrow BR. Vagal esophagomotor nerve function and esophageal motor performance in dogs with congenital idiopathic megaesophagus. Am J Vet Res 1996;57(6):906–13.

[14] Mathews KG, Bunch SK. Vascular liver disease. In: Ettinger SJ, Feldman EC, editors. Text-book of veterinary internal medicine. 6th edition. Philadelphia: WB Saunders; 2005. p. 1453–64.

[15] Center SA, Hornbuckle WE, Hoskins JD. The liver and pancreas. In: Hoskins JD, editor. Veterinary pediatrics. 2nd edition. Philadelphia: WB Saunders; 1990. p. 189–225.

[16] Wrigley RH, Konde LJ, Park RD, et al. Ultrasonographic diagnosis of portocaval shunts in young dogs. J Am Vet Med Assoc 1987;191:421–4.

[17] Breitschwerdt EB, Ochoa R, Barta M, et al. Clinical and laboratory characterization of Ba-senjis with immunoproliferative small intestinal disease. Am J Vet Res 1984;45:267–73.

[18] Hall EJ, Batt RM. Development of a wheat-sensitive enteropathy in Irish setters: biochemical changes. Am J Vet Res 1990;51:983–9.

[19] Hall EJ, Batt RM. Development of a wheat-sensitive enteropathy in Irish setters: morpholog-ical changes. Am J Vet Res 1990;51:978–82.

[20] Fyfe JC, Jezyk PF, Giger U, et al. Inherited selective malabsorption of vitamin B12 in giant schnauzers. J Am Anim Hosp 1989;25:533–9.

[21] Strombeck DR, Guilford WG. The pancreas. In: Small animal gastroenterology. 2nd edi-tion. Davis (CA): Stonegate Publishing; 1990. p. 429–58.

Vet Clin Small Anim 36 (2006) 549–556

VETERINARY CLINICS
SMALL ANIMAL PRACTICE

ELSEVIER SAUNDERS

Pediatric Endocrinology

Deborah S. Greco, DVM, PhD

The Animal Medical Center, 510 East 62nd Street, New York, NY 10021, USA

PITUITARY DISORDERS

Central Diabetes Insipidus

Diabetes insipidus (DI) is a disorder of water metabolism characterized by polyuria, urine of low specific gravity or osmolality, and polydipsia. It is caused by defective secretion of antidiuretic hormone (ADH; central DI) or by the inability of the renal tubule to respond to ADH (nephrogenic DI) [1,2]. Deficiency of ADH (or vasopressin) can be partial or complete. Central DI is characterized by an absolute or relative lack of circulating ADH and is classified as primary (idiopathic and congenital) or secondary. Secondary central DI usually results from head trauma or neoplasia. Central DI and nephrogenic DI are rare disorders.

Central DI may appear at any age, in any breed, and in either gender; however, young animals (6 months of age) are most commonly affected. The major clinical signs of DI are profound polyuria and polydipsia (more than 100 mL/kg/d, normal: 40–70 mL/kg/d), nocturia, and incontinence (usually of several months' duration) [2,3]. The severity of the clinical signs varies, because DI may result from a partial or complete defect in ADH secretion or action. Other less consistent signs include weight loss, because these animals are constantly seeking water, and dehydration.

Routine complete blood cell count (CBC), serum biochemical, and electrolyte profiles are usually normal in animals with DI. Plasma osmolality is often high (>310 mOsm/L) in central or nephrogenic DI as a result of dehydration. Puppies with primary (psychogenic?) polydipsia often exhibit low plasma osmolality (<290 mOsm/L) as a result of overhydration. When abnormalities, such as a slightly increased hematocrit or hypernatremia, are present on initial evaluation, they are usually secondary to dehydration from water restriction by the pet owner. In DI, the results of urinalysis are unremarkable except for the finding of persistently dilute urine (urine specific gravity: 1.004–1.012).

Diagnostic tests to confirm and differentiate central DI, nephrogenic DI, and psychogenic polydipsia include the modified water deprivation test or response to ADH supplementation. The modified water deprivation test is designed to

E-mail address: deborah.greco@amcny.org

0195-5616/06/$ – see front matter
doi:10.1016/j.cvsm.2005.12.005

determine whether endogenous ADH is released in response to dehydration and whether the kidneys can respond to ADH. The more common causes of polyuria and polydipsia should be ruled out before this procedure. Failure to recognize renal failure before water deprivation may lead to an incorrect or inconclusive diagnosis or cause significant patient morbidity. Normal renal concentrating abilities are not present in a puppy until 4 to 6 months of age. Congenital renal dysplasia can cause early signs of renal failure. A simpler way to differentiate between primary or psychogenic polydipsia and DI is to compare water consumption before and 3 to 5 days after desmopressin (DDAVP) administration (2–3 drops nasally or onto the conjunctival sac twice daily); a 50% reduction in water consumption is consistent with a diagnosis of central DI.

Treatment consists of replacement of the deficient hormone (ADH) in the form of desmopressin or DDAVP. Desmopressin, which is used to treat bedwetting in children, is available as a nasal spray; however, the nasal delivery apparatus should be removed before administration to a dog or cat because it can be uncomfortable to them. Two to 3 drops of DDAVP nasally or onto the conjunctival sac twice daily is recommended to control polydipsia and polyuria in most animals with DI [3,4]. It is important to counsel clients about the fact that water deprivation in the untreated patient with central DI can be problematic.

Abnormalities of statural growth

Many pediatric endocrine disorders are manifested as abnormalities of statural growth. Causes of inadequate growth can be divided into two broad categories: intrinsic defects of growing tissues (skeletal dysplasias, chromosomal abnormalities, and dysmorphic dwarfism) and abnormalities in the environment of growing tissues (nutritional, metabolic, environmental, and endocrine). Intrinsic defects of growing tissues include most of the genetic and chromosomal abnormalities that result in growth failure. Genetic disorders may be suspected on the basis of clustering of disease in certain breeds and/or lines of dogs and cats (ie, chondrodystrophy of Alaskan Malamutes). Diagnosis may require pursuing pedigree analysis, genetic testing, or both.

Abnormalities of the environment of growing tissues are the most common and easily identified disorders. A thorough dietary history should reveal an inadequate quantity or quality of feeding. Metabolic disorders, such as portosystemic shunting, pancreatic insufficiency, congenital heart disease, and congenital (dysplastic) renal failure, may be identified by characteristic clinical signs and laboratory data. Endocrine causes of growth retardation include juvenile hypothyroidism, juvenile type I diabetes mellitus, juvenile hyperadrenocorticism, and hypopituitarism.

Endocrine growth abnormalities can be divided into two groups based on the type of dwarfism present. A proportionate dwarf exhibits small stature but precisely the same dimensions as the adult animal; proportionate dwarfism is characteristic of isolated growth hormone (GH) deficiency. In contrast, a disproportionate dwarf has a normal-sized head and trunk with short legs; disproportionate dwarfism is characteristic of hypothyroid- and hyperadrenocorticism-mediated dwarfism (Fig. 1). Other endocrine causes of abnormal growth (ie, juvenile diabetes mellitus) result in subnormal stature (not true dwarfism) and a normally proportioned but emaciated animal.

Pituitary Dwarfism

Pituitary dwarfism results from destruction of the pituitary gland via a neoplastic, degenerative, or anomalous process. It may be associated with decreased production of other pituitary hormones, including thyroid-stimulating hormone (TSH), corticotropin, luteinizing hormone (LH), follicle-stimulating hormone (FSH), and GH. Pituitary dwarfism is most common in German Shepherd Dogs aged 2 to 6 months [5]. Other affected breeds include the Carnelian Bear Dog, Spitz, Miniature Pinscher, and Weimaraner. The disease is inherited as a simple autosomal recessive trait in German Shepherd Dogs and occurs as a result of a cystic Rathke's pouch. The first observable clinical signs of pituitary dwarfism are slow growth noticed in first 2 to 3 months of life and mental retardation, usually manifested as difficulty in house-training. Physical examination findings may include proportionate dwarfism, retained puppy hair coat, hypotonic skin, truncal alopecia, cutaneous hyperpigmentation, infantile genitalia, and delayed dental eruption. Clinicopathologic features include eosinophilia, lymphocytosis, mild normocytic normochromic anemia, hypophosphatemia, and, occasionally, hypoglycemia resulting from secondary adrenal insufficiency. The differential diagnosis includes other causes of stunted growth, such as hypothyroid dwarfism, portosystemic shunt, diabetes mellitus, hyperadrenocorticism, malnutrition, and parasitism. Diagnosis is made by measuring serum GH concentrations (no longer commercially available) or serum somatomedin C (insulin-like growth factor 1 [IGF-1]). The advantage of IGF-1 is that it is not species specific. There is a usually a subnormal response to exogenous TSH and corticotropin stimulation tests; furthermore, endogenous TSH and corticotropin are decreased

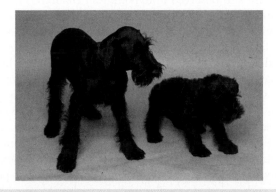

Fig. 1. Disproportionate dwarfism in an 8-month-old hypothyroid Giant Schnauzer puppy compared with a normal littermate.

in affected dogs as a result of panhypopituitarism. The results of a thyrotropin-releasing hormone (TRH) stimulation test would be abnormal as well.

THYROID DISORDERS

Congenital Hypothyroidism

Congenital hypothyroidism is a relatively common endocrine disorder of human infants, resulting in mandatory testing of neonates. In contrast, reports of congenital hypothyroidism in dogs and cats are relatively few. Only 3.6% of the cases of canine hypothyroidism occur in dogs younger than 1 year of age. Congenital hypothyroidism may be caused by aplasia or hypoplasia of the thyroid gland, thyroid ectopia, dyshormonogenesis, maternal goitrogen ingestion, maternal radioactive iodine treatment, iodine deficiency (endemic goiter), autoimmune thyroiditis, hypopituitarism, isolated thyrotropin deficiency, hypothalamic disease, or isolated TRH deficiency [6–12].

Because thyroid hormone secretion is essential for normal postnatal development of the nervous and skeletal systems, congenital hypothyroidism is characterized by disproportionate dwarfism, central and peripheral nervous system abnormalities, and mental deficiency. In addition, many of the signs of adult-onset hypothyroidism, such as lethargy, inappetence, constipation, dermatopathy, and hypothermia, may be observed [11,12].

Congenital hypothyroidism, regardless of cause, results in characteristic historical and physical examination features. Dogs and infants have a history of large birth weight (in human babies, this is the result of prolonged gestation), followed by aberrant and delayed growth. In puppies, the first signs of abnormal growth occur as early as 3 weeks after birth and abnormal body proportions are evident by 8 weeks of age. This is similar to human infants, who are normal at birth but, if undiagnosed, exhibit characteristic signs by 6 to 8 weeks of age [13,14]. Historical findings in hypothyroid puppies, such as lethargy, mental dullness, weak nursing, delayed dental eruption, and abdominal distention, are also observed in hypothyroid children [11,12].

Physical features of hypothyroid dwarfism in children include hypotonia, umbilical hernia, skin mottling, large anterior and posterior fontanels, macroglossia, hoarse cry, distended abdomen, dry skin, jaundice, pallor, slow deep tendon reflex, delayed dental eruption, and hypothermia [13,14]. In dogs with congenital hypothyroidism, hypotonia, macroglossia, distended abdomen, dry skin, delayed dental eruption, and hypothermia have been described (see Fig. 1; Fig. 2) [11,12]. In addition, because dogs develop more rapidly and become weight bearing sooner than human infants, gait abnormalities and disproportionate dwarfism are prominent features of canine congenital hypothyroidism. Midface hypoplasia, a broad nose, and a large protruding tongue are some of the sequelae of untreated hypothyroidism in people. Similar facial features, such as broad maxillas and macroglossia, were observed in affected puppies [11,12]. In human beings, delayed eruption of permanent teeth is observed in untreated congenitally hypothyroid individuals; delayed dental

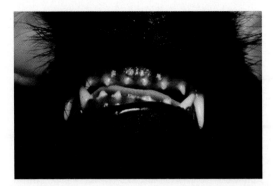

Fig. 2. Delayed dental eruption in an 8-month-old hypothyroid Dwarf Schnauzer puppy.

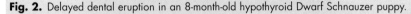

eruption is characteristic of hypothyroid puppies treated after 4 months of age. In human beings and dogs, macroglossia and effusions of the body cavities are the result of myxedematous fluid accumulation. Hypothyroid puppies often exhibit hair coat abnormalities, including retention of the puppy hair coat and thinning of the hair coat.

Thyroid hormone is crucial for proper postnatal development of the nervous system. As a result, a significant number of properly treated and all untreated hypothyroid infants exhibit poor coordination and speech impediments later in life. Delayed treatment often results in low perceptual-motor, visual-spatial, and language scores in children with congenital hypothyroidism. If treatment is delayed beyond 4 to 6 months in human babies, intelligence is irreversibly affected and mental retardation may ensue [13–16]. Mental retardation is also likely in hypothyroid puppies; however, no objective evidence of delayed or aberrant intelligence is available to assess affected pups. Because the bulk of cerebellar development occurs after birth, Purkinje cell growth is also significantly affected by congenital hypothyroidism [17]. In human beings and puppies, if treatment is delayed, signs of cerebellar dysfunction, such as ataxia, are observed. Skeletal abnormalities, such as delayed maturation and epiphyseal dysgenesis, are the hallmark of congenital hypothyroidism. Delayed epiphyseal maturation is observed in the vertebral bodies and long bones of affected puppies. Epiphyseal dysgenesis, which is characterized by a ragged epiphysis with scattered foci of calcification, is observed in human beings and dogs with untreated congenital hypothyroidism (Fig. 3). Normal epiphyseal development proceeds from a single center; however, in hypothyroidism, thyroid deficiency leads to the development of multiple epiphyseal centers, each with its own calcification progression [18]. Disorderly epiphyseal calcification leads to secondary arthropathies in children with untreated congenital hypothyroidism [18].

Clinicopathologic features of congenital hypothyroidism include hypercholesterolemia, hypercalcemia, and mild anemia [19]. Hypercholesterolemia develops in congenital and adult-onset hypothyroidism because of decreased

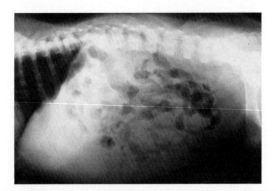

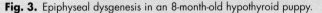

Fig. 3. Epiphyseal dysgenesis in an 8-month-old hypothyroid puppy.

hepatic metabolism and decreased fecal excretion of cholesterol. Hypercalcemia secondary to congenital hypothyroidism is the result of decreased renal clearance and increased gastrointestinal absorption of calcium. Decreased thyroid hormone stimulation of erythropoietic precursors results in a mild normocytic normochromic anemia in some puppies with hypothyroidism [20].

It has been well established that thyroxine is essential for the proper transcription, translation, and secretion of GH by pituitary somatotrophs. In human beings (and most likely in dogs), circulating GH concentrations are high during the first few days after birth but rapidly decrease during the subsequent few weeks to levels just slightly greater than those in adults [21]. In a previously reported case of congenital hypothyroidism, the dog exhibited a blunted GH response to xylazine but had a normal GH response to provocative stimulation after treatment of the hypothyroid state [21].

The diagnosis of congenital hypothyroidism is based on clinical signs, supporting clinicopathologic findings, and thyroid function testing. It is vital to remember that normal puppies aged 5 to 6 weeks have serum total thyroxine (TT4) concentrations two to three times higher than normal adult dogs. Therefore, a serum TT4 of 2.0 μg/dL, which is normal for an adult dog, would be low in a 6-week-old puppy and indicative of thyroid dysfunction. Serum-free thyroxine (FT4) would also be expected to be higher in normal neonatal dogs. Indeed, a recent report of TT4, FT4, total triiodothyronine (TT3), free triiodothyronine (FT3), and reverse T3 (rT3) in puppies from birth to 12 weeks confirmed the suspicion that TT4 and FT4 are high in neonates [22]. At birth, TT4 was within the normal range, but by 1 week of age and until 5 weeks of age, serum TT4 was two to three times the normal adult range. Surprisingly, TT3 and FT3 were much lower in these neonatal puppies, suggesting an inability of neonatal animals to convert T4 to T3 peripherally. The advent of the endogenous canine TSH assay should allow discrimination of primary congenital hypothyroidism from secondary hypothyroidism (TSH deficiency). Puppies with primary hypothyroidism (eg, thyroid dysgenesis, dyshormonogenesis) would be expected to have elevated endogenous TSH concentrations, whereas puppies with TSH deficiency should have subnormal endogenous TSH concentrations. Specific studies on endogenous TSH in neonatal dogs have yet to be performed.

Treatment of congenital hypothyroidism in puppies and kittens is similar to treatment in the adult animal (22–44 µg/kg in the dog and 11 µg/kg brand name L-thyroxine once daily in the cat). Some authors have suggested that hypothyroidism may be a cause of neonatal mortality in puppies; therefore, 1- to 3-week-old pups in high-risk breeds may be screened.

PANCREATIC DISORDERS
Juvenile Diabetes Mellitus
Diabetes mellitus, a common endocrinopathy of adult dogs and cats, is rarely observed in puppies and kittens. All reported cases of diabetes mellitus in juvenile dogs and cats have been type I or insulin-dependent diabetes mellitus (IDDM). Many canine juvenile diabetes mellitus cases, as in human beings, are thought to have a viral cause. Dogs with juvenile diabetes mellitus are usually presented between 3 and 6 months of age. A genetic basis for diabetes mellitus is suspected in the Keeshonden and Samoyed breeds. Predisposed breeds for diabetes mellitus include the Pulik, Cairn Terrier, Miniature Pinscher, Miniature Poodle, Miniature Schnauzer, Dachshund, and Beagle [23].

In young dogs and cats, stunted growth is often associated with diabetes mellitus as a result of calorie deprivation. In dogs, progressive polyuria, polydipsia, and weight loss develop relatively rapidly, usually over a period of several weeks. Another presenting complaint of diabetes mellitus in puppies is the acute onset of blindness caused by cataract formation. Diabetic cataracts can develop rapidly, and the owner may notice that the puppy is suddenly bumping into furniture and other obstacles. The most common physical examination findings are dehydration and muscle wasting or thin body condition. Emaciated diabetic animals may have concurrent underlying disorders, such as exocrine pancreatic insufficiency, particularly those with juvenile-onset diabetes. A diagnosis of diabetes mellitus should be based on the presence of clinical signs compatible with diabetes mellitus and evidence of fasting hyperglycemia and glycosuria.

Treatment of juvenile diabetes mellitus may be challenging. Because these animals are growing rapidly, insulin requirements may change drastically on a daily or weekly basis. The author has had success in treating 12-week-old Greyhound puppies with lente insulin at an initial dose of 0.5 U/kg administered subcutaneously twice daily. Pork lente insulin is recommended. The puppies must be fed three to four times daily; additionally, regular insulin administered subcutaneously at a rate of 0.1 to 0.2 U/kg with meals can be necessary. A growth formulation, rather than high-fiber foods, should be fed to growing puppies and kittens. Caloric requirements should be calculated for a growing animal. Management of concurrent exocrine pancreatic insufficiency requires the use of oral pancreatic extract and, potentially, antibiotics for bacterial overgrowth.

References

[1] Bruyette DS. Polyuria and polydipsia. In: August JR, editor. Consultations in feline internal medicine. Philadelphia: WB Saunders; 1991. p. 227–35.

[2] Nichols CE. Endocrine and metabolic causes of polyuria and polydipsia. In: Kirk RW, Bonagura JD, editors. Current veterinary therapy XI. Philadelphia: WB Saunders; 1992. p. 293–301.

[3] Nichols R. Diabetes insipidus. In: Kirk RW, editor. Current veterinary therapy X. Philadelphia: WB Saunders; 1989. p. 973–8.

[4] Krause KH. The use of desmopressin in diagnosis and treatment of diabetes insipidus in cats. Compend Contin Educ Pract Vet 1987;9:752–5.

[5] Campbell KL. Growth hormone-related disorders in dogs. Compend Contin Educ Pract Vet 1988;10(4):477–82.

[6] Greco DS, Peterson ME, Cho DY. Juvenile-onset hypothyroidism in a dog. J Am Vet Med Assoc 1985;187:948–50.

[7] LaFranchi SH. Hypothyroidism. Pediatr Clin North Am 1979;26:33–51.

[8] Feldman EC, Nelson RW. Hypothyroidism. In: Canine and feline endocrinology and reproduction. 1st edition. Philadelphia: WB Saunders; 1987. p. 55–90.

[9] Milne KL, Hayes HM. Epidemiologic features of canine hypothyroidism. Cornell Vet 1981;71:3–14.

[10] Chastain CB, McNeil SV, Graham CL, et al. Congenital hypothyroidism in a dog due to an iodide organification defect. Am J Vet Res 1983;44:1257–65.

[11] Medleau L, Eigenmann JE, Saunders HM, et al. Congenital hypothyroidism in a dog. J Am Anim Hosp Assoc 1985;21:341–3.

[12] Robinson WF, Shaw SE, Stanley B, et al. Congenital hypothyroidism in Scottish Deerhound puppies. Aust Vet J 1988;65:386–9.

[13] Kenny FM, Klein AH, Augustin AV, et al. Sporadic cretinism. In: Fisher DA, Gurrow GN, editors. Perinatal thyroid physiology and disease. New York: Raven Press; 1975. p. 73–8.

[14] Fisher DA. Medical management of suspected cases of congenital hypothyroidism. In: Burrow GN, editor. Neonatal thyroid screening. New York: Raven Press; 1980. p. 237–44.

[15] Sawin CT. Hypothyroidism. Med Clin North Am 1985;69:989–1004.

[16] Moschini L, Costa P, Marinelli E, et al. Longitudinal assessment of children with congenital hypothyroidism detected by neonatal screening. Helv Paediatr Acta 1986;41:415–24.

[17] Noguchi T, Sugisaki T. Hypomyelination in the cerebrum of the congenitally hypothyroid mouse (hyt). J Neurochem 1984;42:891–3.

[18] Wilkins L. Epiphyseal dysgenesis associated with hypothyroidism. Am J Dis Child 1941;61:13–34.

[19] Tau C, Garagedian M, Farriaux JP, et al. Hypercalcemia in infants with congenital hypothyroidism and its relation to vitamin D and thyroid hormones. J Pediatr 1986;109:808–14.

[20] Cline MJ, Berlin NI. Erythropoiesis and red cell survival in the hypothyroid dog. Am J Physiol 1963;204:415–8.

[21] Wood DF, Franklyn JA, Docherty K. The effect of thyroid hormones on growth hormone gene expression in vivo in rats. J Endocrinol 1987;112:459–63.

[22] Casal ML, Zerbe CA, Jezyk PF, et al. Thyroid profiles in healthy puppies from birth to 12 weeks of age [abstract]. Proc Amer Coll Vet Int Med 1994;989.

[23] Greco DS, Chastain CB. Endocrine and metabolic systems. In: Hoskins JW, editor. Veterinary pediatrics. 3rd edition. Philadelphia: WB Saunders; 2001. p. 353–5.

Vet Clin Small Anim 36 (2006) 557–572

VETERINARY CLINICS
SMALL ANIMAL PRACTICE

ELSEVIER
SAUNDERS

Topics in Pediatric Dermatology

Terry Nagle, BVSc, MACVSc

VCA–Sacramento Animal Medical Group, 4990 Manzanita Avenue, Carmichael, CA 95608, USA

Skin conditions of puppies and kittens include several infectious conditions, such as ectoparasites and dermatophytosis. In the case of impetigo, demodicosis, dermatophytosis, and papillomatosis, this may be at least partially attributable to their immune systems not being fully developed or their acquired immunity lacking experience with the organisms involved. The function of the skin as a barrier may also not be fully developed in pediatric patients.

Hereditary and congenital skin problems are usually manifest, and therefore often detected, at an early age. Some conditions, such as ichthyosis, acrodermatitis, and primary immune deficiencies, are attributable to a defect in the structure or function of the skin, whereas dermatomyositis is thought to involve a genetic predisposition that produces disease when combined with an environmental insult.

Young animals may be more prone to toxicity from medications, and labels should be read carefully for age limits. Husbandry factors, including nutrition, ectoparasites, temperature and humidity, cleaning products, and bedding, should be considered in the pathogenesis of disease processes. Fleas are still a common problem despite recent improvements in flea control and can be debilitating in young animals because of blood loss. Lack of compliance, only treating some animals in the household, not treating environmental contamination with juvenile flea stages, and substitution of less effective, and often more toxic, over-the-counter flea control products are the most common causes of flea infestations and toxicity.

DEMODICOSIS
Cause and Pathogenesis
Demodex canis mites are part of the normal flora of dogs residing in the hair follicles and sebaceous glands. They are acquired only by direct maternal-neonatal contact in the first few days of life, except under experimental conditions [1]. A hereditary predisposition to overgrowth of *D canis* mites has been observed, with an autosomal recessive mode suggested [2]. The immune

E-mail address: terry.nagle@vcamail.com

0195-5616/06/$ – see front matter
doi:10.1016/j.cvsm.2006.01.001

deficiency seems to be a specific T-cell defect; thus, affected dogs may not have other signs of immune deficiency. The Pit Bull Terrier may be overrepresented. Other *Demodex* spp have been described in dogs and cats but are not commonly a cause of disease in pediatric patients.

Clinical Presentation

Demodicosis produces a folliculitis with patches of erythema and alopecia, especially on the head and paws, where puppies contact their dams during suckling. Most cases are not pruritic, although secondary bacterial pyoderma may produce pruritus.

The disease is traditionally classified as juvenile onset or adult onset. Juvenile-onset demodicosis is subdivided into a localized form (no more than five lesions or one region of the body) and a generalized form (more than five lesions or one region of the body or any paw involvement), although there is some overlap between the two [2,3].

Differential Diagnosis

Bacterial pyoderma, demodicosis, and dermatophytosis should be considered in any folliculitis. Multiple deep skin scrapings to produce blood should be performed and examined under a ×10 objective lens. A mixing spatula dipped in mineral oil may be used rather than a scalpel blade. Closing the iris on the condenser to increase contrast makes the translucent cigar-shaped *Demodex* mites (Fig. 1) easier to observe. A biopsy may be required if severe scarring is present or in certain breeds, such as the Shar Pei, possibly because of long hair follicles, as well as reportedly in the Old English Sheepdog or Scottish Terrier [2,3]. The identification of any *D canis* mites on scraping should be considered significant, especially in the presence of clinical signs, and further scrapings should be performed to identify the extent of the disease accurately. Demodicosis can be easily

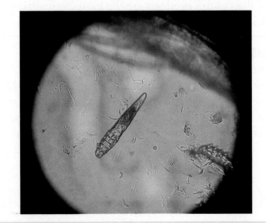

Fig. 1. *Demodex canis* mite from a dog.

missed unless multiple scrapings that produce capillary bleeding are performed and examined carefully.

Therapy

Most cases of juvenile-onset localized demodicosis resolve without miticidal therapy over a period of 3 months. Supportive therapy includes attending to any nutritional or husbandry concerns and treatment of secondary pyoderma. Benzyl peroxide shampoo may be used to flush the follicles and assist in resolution of bacterial folliculitis. Some cases of juvenile-onset generalized demodicosis resolve without miticidal therapy. If clinical signs are still present after 3 months of supportive therapy, then miticidal therapy is probably indicated.

Amitraz is labeled for the treatment of generalized demodicosis in dogs as a rinse at 0.025% given 14 days apart for three to six treatments. Current data do not support the use of amitraz in localized demodicosis, and safety has not established for dogs less than 4 months of age [4]. Additional stress should be avoided for 24 hours after dipping. Higher success rates have been achieved with higher concentrations or frequencies of application, although this may be an off-label use. Amitraz may be toxic to animals and human beings who are diabetic or receiving monoamine oxidase inhibitors or selective serotonin reuptake inhibitors.

A recent review found good evidence for the use of weekly to biweekly rinses with amitraz at 0.025% to 0.05% or with oral ivermectin at a dose of 300 to 600 µg/kg/d, oral milbemycin oxime at a dose of 2 mg/kg/d, and oral moxidectin at a dose of 400 µg/kg/d. The oral macrolides are often started at a lower dose and gradually increased to look for signs of toxicity, although the onset of toxicity may be tardive. One protocol involves gradually increasing the dose of ivermectin given each day from 50 to 100 to 200 µg/kg and then to 300 µg/kg to identify ivermectin-sensitive dogs. Ivermectin has a long half-life; thus, cumulative toxicity is still possible. Clients should sign a consent form for off-label use of this product [3].

There was good evidence against the use of ronnel (because of the risk of toxicity) and levamisole (because of the lack of clinical efficacy) in dogs as well as for the use of weekly 2% lime sulfur dips for demodicosis in cats [3].

Miticidal therapy should be continued until two consecutive negative scrapings are obtained 4 to 6 weeks apart (remission), with negative meaning not a single live or dead mite. After remission, dogs should be observed closely for 12 months for any clinical signs of recurrence, such as alopecia or scaling, and deep skin scrapings should be performed.

Ivermectin is not licensed for treatment of demodicosis in dogs and should not be used in herding breeds (Collies, Shetland Sheepdogs, Old English Sheepdogs, and Australian Shepherds) or their crosses, and adverse effects have been observed in other breeds. A polymerase chain reaction (PCR) test is currently available for the multidrug resistance gene responsible for ivermectin sensitivity in Collies and related breeds (Veterinary Clinical Pharmacology Laboratory, Washington State University, Pullman, WA; VCPL@vetmed.wsu.edu).

Milbemycin at a dose of 1 to 2 mg/kg/d has been found to have a low risk of toxicity in the ivermectin-sensitive breeds.

Prevention
Dogs that recover from localized demodicosis without miticidal therapy may be used for breeding unless there is a familial history of demodicosis. Animals that develop generalized demodicosis and their siblings should not be used for breeding [2].

CHEYLETIELLOSIS
Cause and Pathogenesis
Three species of surface-living mites may cause scaling pruritic dermatitis of young animals. *Cheyletiella yasguri*, *C blakei*, and *C parasitovorax* are traditionally associated with dogs, cats, and rabbits, respectively, but the mites are not highly host specific and may cause transient signs in human beings in areas of direct contact with an infested animal [2].

Clinical Presentation
Dorsal scaling with variable erythema and pruritus are reported, and signs may increase with time. Cats with cheyletiellosis may be presented with miliary dermatitis or as overgroomers. Subclinical carrier status is possible.

Differential Diagnosis
Superficial skin scrapings, acetate tape preparation, and fecal floatation may be used to reveal large mites with combs rather than claws and hooked mouth parts. Mites may not be detectable in some cases. *Cheyletiella* eggs are large and loosely attached to hairs rather than firmly cemented as are louse eggs.

Therapy
All dogs and cats (and rabbits) in the household should be treated, and the environment should be treated. Lime sulfur dips can be used weekly in young puppies and kittens. Selamectin or fipronil at label doses, ivermectin at 200 to 300 µg/kg administered subcutaneously, or milbemycin at 1 to 2 mg/kg administered orally, repeated twice at 14-day intervals, is usually effective. An environmental flea control spray may be used as directed on the environment, and bedding should be washed and dried and fomites discarded [5–7].

Prevention
Quarantine of new animals and prevention of sharing of fomites should reduce the incidence of cheyletiellosis.

DERMATOPHYTOSIS
Cause and Pathogenesis
Dermatophytes are fungi that can infect keratinized tissues, such as the hair, claws, stratum corneum, and feathers. *Microsporum canis*, *M gypseum*, and *Trichophyton* mentagrophytes are the most common dermatophytes detected in dogs and cats. Dermatophytosis is more common in warm and humid environments

and in young, sick, debilitated, and old animals. Long-haired cats are commonly considered to be more prone to dermatophytosis and subclinical carrier status. Dermatophytosis is a zoonosis and may occur more commonly in children or immunosuppressed persons [8,9].

Clinical Presentation

Dermatophytosis in young patients usually presents as folliculitis, but clinical signs can be variable, especially in cats. Puppies and kittens may be presented with patches of alopecia (Fig. 2), possibly with erythema, papules, pustules, scale, or crusting, and kittens may have crusted papules. The degree of inflammation may be inversely proportional to the number of fungal organisms present. Pruritus ranges from nonexistent to severe.

Differential Diagnosis

Hairs infected with *M canis* may fluoresce under a Wood's lamp, but the lamp should be warmed to operating temperature for 5 to 10 minutes and hairs exposed for 3 to 5 minutes. False-positive and false-negative results are possible. The Wood's lamp may be used as a screening test, and hairs that fluoresce should be submitted for culture. Direct examination of hairs in mineral oil may reveal fungal hyphae or spores, but sensitivity is increased by the use of a clearing agent, such potassium hydroxide or chlorphenolac. Fungal culture is considered the "gold standard." Because of the potential for zoonosis (Fig. 3) and accusations of infection before purchase, hairs, and ideally scale, should be submitted for fungal culture and identification of dermatophyte species by an accredited laboratory in all cases.

Therapy

A recent review suggests that the best treatment may be a combination of clipping of the hair coat, twice-weekly topical antifungal therapy, concurrent systemic antifungal therapy, and environmental decontamination. Treatment

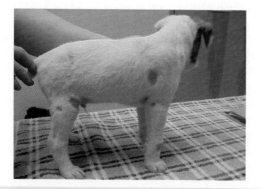

Fig. 2. Jack Russell Terrier puppy with patches of alopecia and erythema attributable to *Microsporum canis* infection.

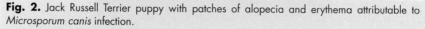

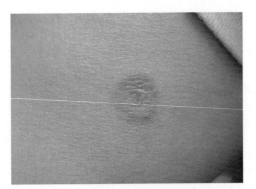
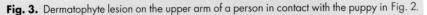

Fig. 3. Dermatophyte lesion on the upper arm of a person in contact with the puppy in Fig. 2.

should be continued until two or three consecutive negative fungal cultures are obtained at weekly or biweekly intervals [9].

Because of the risk of carrier status, all cats should be treated with systemic therapy; nevertheless, topical therapy and environmental decontamination are still required. Dermatophytosis may be self-limiting in puppies. Single lesions in puppies may be treated with topical therapy and environmental decontamination, but systemic therapy may be added for nonresponsive cases.

Topical Therapy

Topical therapy may include lime sulfur dips at a ratio of 1:16, 0.2% enilconazole rinses, or shampoo containing a combination of 2% miconazole and 2% chlorhexidine. Lime sulfur dip is labeled for use in puppies and kittens at a 1:32 dilution, but enilconazole is not labeled for small animal use in the United States. Spot treatment for individual lesions may also include 1% clotrimazole creams or lotions or 2% miconazole cream or lotion.

Systemic Therapy

Microsized griseofulvin may be used at a dose of 50 mg/kg/d (10–15 mg/kg/d for the ultramicrosized form) administered orally. Absorption is increased by administration with fatty food. Concerns have been expressed about bone marrow suppression in feline immunodeficiency virus (FIV)-positive cats and, anecdotally, of increased risk of adverse effects in oriental breeds [8].

Itraconazole at a dose of 5 to 10 mg/kg/d may be used, and the pediatric (10 mg/mL) oral suspension is convenient for small patients. Additionally, the β-glycan base used in this solution provides superior bioavailability. Other dosing regimens have been described. Terbinafine has also been used and is well tolerated by dogs and cats at a dose of 30 to 40 mg/kg administered orally every 24 hours.

Environmental Decontamination

Treatment of surfaces with dilute sodium hypochlorite is effective but can be irritating to skin and eyes. Fomites should be treated or removed.

Prevention

Fungal culture using the McKenzie toothbrush technique before purchase can be performed before introduction to households with children or immunosuppressed persons, but final results take 3 weeks. A new toothbrush is passed through the coat, and any hairs removed are submitted for fungal culture. Quarantine of new introductions or animals returning from shows or stud visits, regular decontamination of transport cages and grooming equipment, and avoidance of repeated use of grooming equipment for multiple animals can reduce spread of dermatophytes. Dermatophyte spores may remain infectious for many months.

IMPETIGO

Cause and Pathogenesis

Impetigo is typically caused by infection with *Staphylococcus* organisms. The infections may be secondary to husbandry problems but may occur in cases with apparently excellent husbandry and nutrition [10].

Clinical Presentation

Impetigo presents as superficial pustules that are not associated with hair follicles, usually on areas of skin with little hair, such as the ventral abdomen and axilla.

Differential Diagnosis

Cocci bacteria are found in smears from pustule contents.

THERAPY AND PREVENTION

Any husbandry or nutritional problems should be addressed, and affected areas may be washed gently in an antibacterial shampoo, such as chlorhexidine or ethyl lactate. Oral antibiotics are not usually required but may be used in some cases.

CUTANEOUS PAPILLOMAS

Cause and Pathogenesis

A number of different clinical presentations in dogs are reported or suspected to involve papillomaviruses. More recent research has been conducted on a molecular basis than on clinical appearance. Papillomavirus is quite stable in the environment and can survive for up to 63 days at 4°C to 8°C or for 6 hours at 37°C. The incubation period is 1 to 2 months [11].

Clinical Presentation

Canine oral papillomatosis produces multiple lesions in the oral cavity and on the head of dogs. The lesions begin as smooth white papules or plaques and progress to whitish-gray hyperkeratotic lesions that may cover much of the face and mouth [12]. Papillomas have also been observed under the tongue of cats [13].

Differential Diagnosis

Histopathologic findings can be used to differentiate papillomas from other epidermal tumors.

Therapy and Prevention

Spontaneous remission usually occurs in a few months. Surgical debridement or cryosurgery may be required if the masses interfere with eating or hygiene. Vaccines and immunomodulating drugs have not been documented to speed resolution of lesions. Although a vaccine has been shown to be protective, cutaneous neoplasms have been reported with a live vaccine and no vaccine is commercially available for dogs [11,12,14–16].

CANINE JUVENILE CELLULITIS
Cause and Pathogenesis

Hereditary factors are suspected in the pathogenesis of canine juvenile cellulitis because of a breed predisposition, including Golden Retrievers, Gordon Setters, and Dachshunds, although not all puppies in a litter may be affected. Attempts to transfer the disease by inoculation or to detect infectious agents have not been successful [17].

Clinical Presentation

Canine juvenile cellulitis is most commonly seen in puppies less than 12 weeks of age, although it may rarely occur in young adults. The initial lesions may be small areas of erythema or papules on the face, including the eyelids, lips, and medial aspects of the pinnae, and marked edema of the face (Figs. 4–6). Submandibular lymphadenopathy is usually present [15]. The lesions may progress rapidly to draining fistulae and crusts, and other peripheral lymph nodes may be enlarged. Affected puppies may be anorexic, pyrexic, or lethargic, and joint pain may be present. Secondary bacterial pyoderma may occur, but unbroken nodules have been found to be sterile [18].

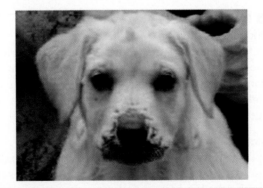

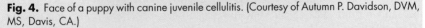

Fig. 4. Face of a puppy with canine juvenile cellulitis. (Courtesy of Autumn P. Davidson, DVM, MS, Davis, CA.)

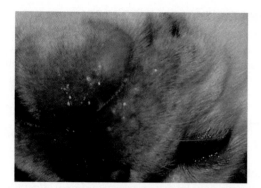

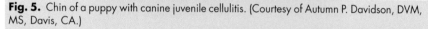

Fig. 5. Chin of a puppy with canine juvenile cellulitis. (Courtesy of Autumn P. Davidson, DVM, MS, Davis, CA.)

Differential Diagnosis

Demodicosis must be eliminated before immunosuppressive therapy is commenced. Severe pyoderma or a cutaneous adverse drug reaction may produce similar signs. Cytology shows pyogranulomatous inflammation without organisms, and pyogranulomatous inflammation predominated by epithelioid macrophages is observed on histopathologic examination of the skin and lymph nodes [17].

Therapy

Prednisone at a dose of 2 mg/kg/d administered orally should be given until the inflammation has resolved so as to decrease the incidence of scarring, and the dose should then be tapered. Concurrent treatment with antibiotics, such as cephalosporins and prednisone, is effective in treating secondary bacterial infection [18]. Griseofulvin has also been used [19].

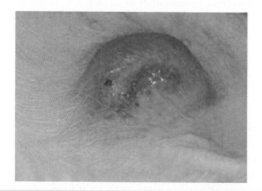

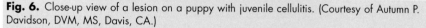

Fig. 6. Close-up view of a lesion on a puppy with juvenile cellulitis. (Courtesy of Autumn P. Davidson, DVM, MS, Davis, CA.)

PRIMARY KERATINIZATION DISORDERS
Cause and Pathogenesis
An inherited disorder of keratinization (seborrhea) has been reported in American Cocker Spaniels, English Springer Spaniels, West Highland White Terriers, and Basset Hounds, and clinical signs may be noted as early as 10 weeks of age. Irish Setters, German Shepherd Dogs, Dachshunds, Doberman Pinschers, Shar Peis, and Labrador Retrievers may also be affected.

A primary seborrhea has been reported in Persian kittens as early as a few days of life, and therapy has not been successful [20].

Clinical Presentation
Accumulations of scale may be dry or greasy and may affect the ears and claws. Pruritus may also be present. Secondary superficial pyoderma and *Malassezia* dermatitis are common and often recurrent.

Differential Diagnosis
Primary seborrhea is a diagnosis of exclusion, but in dogs less than 1 year of age, the differential diagnosis includes demodicosis, cheyletiellosis, nutritional imbalances, ichthyosis, and epidermal dysplasia.

Therapy
Shampoos may be used to assist in management, but potent products may stimulate keratin production further. Retinoids have had varying success in cases of primary seborrhea. Oral prednisolone at a dose of 1 to 2 mg/kg/d may be used to control seborrhea and then tapered slowly to an alternate-day maintenance dose. Prednisolone increases the risk of secondary infections, and long-term therapy is required.

ICHTHYOSIS
Cause and Pathogenesis
Ichthyosis is used to refer to a number of clinical keratinization disorders in human beings, including epidermolytic hyperkeratosis (caused by dominant mutations affecting keratins 1 and 10) and lamellar ichthyosis. Conditions resembling ichthyosis have been reported and described in dogs and one cat, and, recently, one presentation resembling epidermolytic hyperkeratosis has been found to be a recessive trait affecting keratin 10 in a family of Norfolk Terriers [20–23].

Clinical Presentation
Ichthyosis has been reported in many breeds, and the clinical presentation may vary, because the term may refer to a number of conditions with different causes. Affected West Highland White Terriers and Jack Russell Terriers have reportedly been affected at birth with tightly adherent scales and feathered projections of keratin. The author has seen cases in Golden Retrievers as well as in an American Bulldog (Figs. 7 and 8) Affected Norfolk Terriers

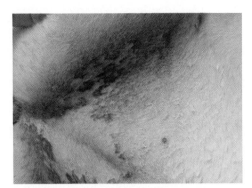

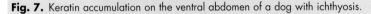

Fig. 7. Keratin accumulation on the ventral abdomen of a dog with ichthyosis.

have generalized pigmented hyperkeratosis with epidermal fragility. Secondary infections may develop.

Differential Diagnosis

A biopsy can be used to confirm the diagnosis and usually shows a prominent granular layer and high mitotic index among the keratinocytes. Electron microscopy and molecular biology techniques are now being used to provide more specific information.

Therapy

Because more potent shampoos may stimulate keratin production, the mildest shampoo possible should be used. Hydration of the skin with Humilac spray (Virbac, Fort Worth, Texas) or a 50% solution of propylene glycol in water may be applied frequently. Retinoid drugs (isotretinoin at a dose of 1–2 mg/kg administered orally every 12 hours or etretinate at a dose of 2.5 mg/kg administered orally every 24 hours) have been reported as beneficial in the

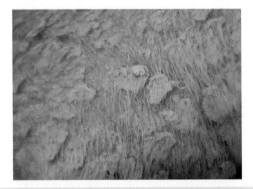

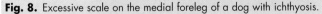

Fig. 8. Excessive scale on the medial foreleg of a dog with ichthyosis.

treatment of ichthyosis in dogs, but the response may take 6 months. Etretinate is no longer available, but acitretin at a dose of 0.5 to 1.0 mg/kg administered orally every 24 hours has been suggested as a replacement. Owners should be advised of the incurable nature the condition. Secondary infections, such as *Malassezia* dermatitis, may be recurrent or persistent, and many affected animals are euthanized.

Prevention

Affected dogs or cats as well as their siblings and parents should not be used for breeding, because an autosomal recessive mode of inheritance has been confirmed in Norfolk Terriers and is suspected in many other breeds.

FAMILIAL CANINE DERMATOMYOSITIS

Cause and Pathogenesis

Familial canine dermatomyositis is a hereditary inflammatory condition affecting the skin and muscles of Collies, Shetland Sheepdogs, and Beauceron Shepherds that has also been reported in the Kuvasz, Welsh Corgi, and other breeds [20,24].

Clinical Presentation

Clinical signs may appear as early as 7 weeks of age, and the rate of progression of skin lesions is variable, but the extent of skin lesions is usually evident by 12 months of age.

Primary vesicles occur in areas of mechanical trauma, such as the face (Fig. 9), ears, tail tip (Fig. 10), digits, and carpal and tarsal regions (Fig. 11), but erythema scale and crusting are usually noted. The claws may also be affected, and secondary bacterial folliculitis may develop.

Myositis usually develops months after dermatologic lesions and commonly affects the muscles of mastication. Megaesophagus and dysphagia may develop in severe cases and may lead to aspiration pneumonia.

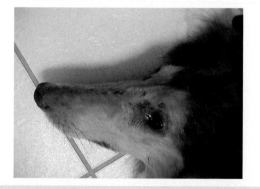

Fig. 9. Areas of alopecia on the face of a Rough Collie with dermatomyositis.

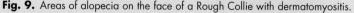

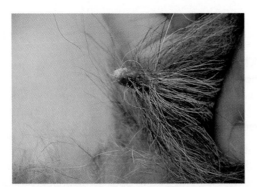

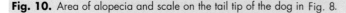
Fig. 10. Area of alopecia and scale on the tail tip of the dog in Fig. 8.

Differential Diagnosis
A skin biopsy is often used to support the diagnosis, and muscle biopsies or electromyographic studies may also be performed.

Therapy
Trauma and solar radiation aggravate dermatomyositis lesions. Prednisolone at a dose of 1 to 2 mg/kg administered orally every 24 hours produces a response in most skin signs but may produce muscle wasting, which compounds muscle damage.

Pentoxifylline at a dose of 25 mg/kg administered orally every 12 hours for 3 months produced a complete response in 4 of 10 dogs with dermatomyositis and a partial response in 6, although prednisone may be required in the initial management of severe cases because of the time delay of pentoxifylline [25]. The long-term prognosis for severe cases is guarded.

Supplementation with vitamin E at a dose of 200 to 800 IU/d administered orally and essential fatty acids may reduce the severity of skin lesions.

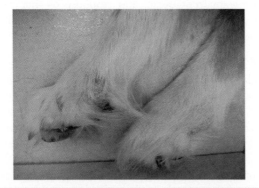

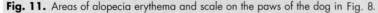
Fig. 11. Areas of alopecia erythema and scale on the paws of the dog in Fig. 8.

Prevention
Affected dogs and their siblings should not be used for breeding.

ACRODERMATITIS OF BULL TERRIERS
Cause and Pathogenesis
Acrodermatitis is an autosomal recessive condition resulting in a lethal syndrome in Bull Terriers; it resembles conditions in human beings and cattle and involves defective zinc and copper metabolism [20,26].

Clinical Presentation
Puppies have dull brittle coats with lighter pigmentation and high-arched hard palates that affect chewing and lead to poor growth. Splayed paws and cracked paw pads as well as skin lesions develop as early as 6 weeks of age. Aggression and subsequent lethargy may develop, and the mean survival time is 7 months. *Malassezia* dermatitis is common, and *Candida* dermatitis has also been reported [20,27].

Differential Diagnosis
Skin biopsies are used to confirm the diagnosis.

Therapy
Treatment for secondary bacterial or *Malassezia* dermatitis does not prevent recurrence, and supplementation with zinc has not been useful [20]. Siblings may also have zinc-responsive dermatosis.

Prevention
Affected animals as well as their parents and siblings should not be used for breeding.

PRIMARY IMMUNODEFICIENCIES
Congenital defects in immunity producing skin lesions have been reported in a variety of breeds of dog, including the Irish Setter, Brittany Spaniel, Doberman Pinscher, Weimaraner, Bull Terrier, Basset Hound, Pomeranian, Cocker Spaniel, and Collie. Skin infections develop without apparent cause or are disproportional to an apparent cause, and response to therapy may be slow. Poorly responsive pyoderma in German Shepherd Dogs usually does not manifest until adulthood [10].

SKIN BIOPSY TECHNIQUE
Samples of skin for histopathologic examination may be required for diagnosis of some conditions. Multiple samples should be taken whenever possible from a range of lesions from all stages of the disease process. Primary lesions should be included whenever possible and taken before glucocorticoids are administered. Normal skin cannot be easily identified after fixation in formalin; thus, samples should not contain large amounts of normal tissue. The skin should not be clipped or surgically prepared apart from gentle removal of excessive hair by scissors if required. Critical information may be contained in the uppermost layers or attached crusts, some of which is lost in processing anyway.

Pediatric patients may require anesthesia or sedation. If local anesthetic is used, it should be injected under but not into the skin; immediately afterward, instruments and paperwork can prepared to allow time for the drug to take effect. Local anesthetic containing epinephrine should not be used on extremities, and the total dose of lidocaine for puppies or kittens should not exceed 0.5 mL because this may provoke seizures, especially if injected in the head region [28].

A circular biopsy punch is often used and always should be rotated in the same direction gently to provide steady pressure until the skin has been penetrated. The punch is then removed, and the sample is gently extracted with forceps and detached from the subcutis with iris scissors. The sample should be rolled gently on a gauze square to remove excess blood and then placed in 10% buffered neutral formalin, which may be supplied by the laboratory. Instruments should never touch the fixative so as to avoid formalin transfer to the patient. A 6-mm punch is usually preferred, although a 4-mm punch is sometimes sufficient. A single suture is usually placed in each site. A detailed history should be supplied, including any differential diagnosis, and samples should be submitted to a histopathologist with specific training in dermatohistopathology. Contacting the laboratory before the sample is submitted may be useful.

References

[1] Caswell JL, Yager JA, Barta JR, et al. Establishment of Demodex canis on canine skin engrafted onto SCID-beige mice. J Parasitol 1996;82(6):911–5.

[2] Scott DW, Miller WH Jr, Griffin CE. Parasitic skin diseases. In: Muller and Kirk's small animal dermatology. 6th edition. Philadelhia: WB Saunders; 2001. p. 423–516.

[3] Mueller RS. Treatment protocols for demodicosis: an evidence-based review. Vet Dermatol 2004;15(2):75–89.

[4] Product Information. Mitaban. Kalamazoo (MI): Pharmacia and Upjohn; 1998.

[5] Scarampella F, Pollmeier M, Visser M, et al. Efficacy of fipronil in the treatment of feline cheyletiellosis. Vet Parasitol 2005;129(3–4):333–9.

[6] Chailleux N, Paradis M. Efficacy of selamectin in the treatment of naturally acquired cheyletiellosis in cats. Can Vet J 2002;43(10):767–70.

[7] Curtis CF. Current trends in the treatment of Sarcoptes, Cheyletiella and Otodectes mite infestations in dogs and cats. Vet Dermatol 2004;15(2):108–14.

[8] Scott DW, Miller WH Jr, Griffin CE. Muller and Kirk's small animal dermatology. 6th edition. Philadelphia: WB Saunders; 2001. p. 336–422.

[9] Moriello KA. Treatment of dermatophytosis in dogs and cats: review of published studies. Vet Dermatol 2004;15(2):99–107.

[10] Scott DW, Miller WH Jr, Griffin CE. Bacterial skin diseases. In: Muller and Kirk's small animal dermatology. 6th edition. Philadelhia: WB Saunders; 2001. p. 274–335.

[11] Nichols PK, Stanley MA. Canine papillomatosis—a centenary review. J Comp Pathol 1999;120(3):219–33.

[12] Scott DW, Miller WH Jr, Griffin CE. Viral, rickettsial, and protozoal skin diseases. In: Muller and Kirk's small animal dermatology. 6th edition. Philadelhia: WB Saunders; 2001. p. 517–42.

[13] Sundberg JP, Van Ranst M, Montali R, et al. Feline papillomas and papillomaviruses. Vet Pathol 2000;37(1):1–10.

[14] Bregman CL, Hirth RS, Sundberg JP, et al. Cutaneous neoplasms in dogs associated with canine oral papillomavirus vaccine. Vet Pathol 1987;24(6):477–87.

[15] Bell JA, Sundberg JP, Ghim SJ, et al. A formalin-inactivated vaccine protects against mucosal papillomavirus infection: a canine model. Pathobiology 1994;63(4):194–8.

[16] Wall M, Calvert CA. Canine viral papillomatosis. In: Greene CE, editor. Infectious diseases of the dog and cat. 3rd edition. St. Louis (MO): Elsevier Saunders; 2006. p. 73–8.

[17] Reimann KA, Evans MG, Chalifoux LV, et al. Clinicopathologic characterization of canine juvenile cellulitis. Vet Pathol 1989;26(6):499–504.

[18] White SD, Rosychuk RA, Stewart LJ, et al. Juvenile cellulitis in dogs: 15 cases (1979–1988). J Am Vet Med Assoc 1989;195(11):1609–11.

[19] Shibata K, Nagata M. Efficacy of griseofulvin for juvenile cellulitis in dogs. Vet Dermatol 2004;15(Suppl 1):26.

[20] Scott DW, Miller WH Jr, Griffin CE. Congenital and hereditary defects. In: Muller and Kirk's small animal dermatology. 6th edition. Philadelhia: WB Saunders; 2001. p. 913–1004.

[21] Muller GH. Ichthyosis in two dogs. J Am Vet Med Assoc 1976;169(12):1313–6.

[22] Mecklenburg L, Hetzel U, Ueberschar S. Epidermolytic ichthyosis in a dog: clinical, histopathological, immunohistochemical and ultrastructural findings. J Comp Pathol 2000; 122(4):307–11.

[23] Credille KM, Barnhart KF, Minor JS, et al. Mild recessive epidermolytic hyperkeratosis associated with a novel keratin 10 donor splice-site mutation in a family of Norfolk terrier dogs. Br J Dermatol 2005;153(1):51–8.

[24] Hargis AM, Haupt KH, Hegreberg GA, et al. Familial canine dermatomyositis. Initial characterization of the cutaneous and muscular lesions. Am J Pathol 1984;116(2):234–44.

[25] Rees CA, Boothe DM. Therapeutic response to pentoxifylline and its active metabolites in dogs with familial canine dermatomyositis. Vet Ther 2003;4(3):234–41.

[26] Jezyk PF, Haskins ME, MacKay-Smith WE, et al. Lethal acrodermatitis in bull terriers. J Am Vet Med Assoc 1986;188(8):833–9.

[27] McEwan NA. Malassezia and Candida infections in bull terriers with lethal acrodermatitis. J Small Anim Pract 2001;42(6):291–7.

[28] Scott DW, Miller WH Jr, Griffin CE. Diagnostic methods. In: Muller and Kirk's small animal dermatology. 6th edition. Philadelhia: WB Saunders; 2001. p. 71–206.

Vet Clin Small Anim 36 (2006) 573–606

VETERINARY CLINICS
SMALL ANIMAL PRACTICE

Disorders of Sexual Differentiation in Puppies and Kittens: A Diagnostic and Clinical Approach

Stefano Romagnoli, DVM, MS, PhD[a],*,
Donald H. Schlafer, DVM, MS, PhD[b]

[a]Department of Veterinary Clinical Sciences, University of Padua, Agripolis I-35020,
Legnaro (Padua), Italy
[b]Department of Biomedical Sciences, Cornell University, Ithaca, NY, USA

A s in all domestic mammals, sexual differentiation in dogs and cats starts early in the embryonic period prenatally and continues into early postnatal life. The result of such a process is, however, not evident until after puberty, a time when the entire reproductive system undergoes significant changes. Normality of sexual differentiation is difficult to observe in neonates of small animals, with the only gender difference being a slightly longer anogenital distance in male (13–15 mm) versus female (7–8 mm) animals. From the first few weeks of life until puberty, deviations from normality that generally cannot be detected by owners include ambiguity of external genitalia and, in male animals, failure to complete testicular descent. After puberty, internal and external genitalia grow and start functioning, allowing owners and breeders to detect potential deviations from normality in the reproduction patterns of their dogs and cats. Early diagnosis of all such conditions can spare breeders the time and effort devoted to raising an animal that may turn out to be unsuitable for becoming part of the reproductive stock and may spare owners the concern for a pet whose health may be unnecessarily threatened by failing to remove a malformed reproductive system early in life. This article reviews the incidence, clinical and gross anatomic features, and diagnostic approaches that veterinarians can use to address inborn errors of the reproductive system of dogs and cats, highlighting those malformations that bear clinical relevance and may become manifest from birth until puberty.

The review of the vast body of international literature available on this topic has greatly benefited from the material published by Johnston, Root-Kustrit, and Olson in 2001 (*Canine and Feline Theriogenology*, edited by WB Saunders), whose elegant literature reviews on related topics have provided inspiration for this chapter.

*Corresponding author. E-mail address: stefano.romagnoli@unipd.it (S. Romagnoli).

GONADAL ABNORMALITIES
Ovarian Abnormalities

Absence of the Y chromosome, and therefore of its sex-determining gene called *Sry*, leads to differentiation of the undifferentiated embryonic gonad into an ovary [1,2]. Congenital abnormalities of the ovary include agenesis (also referred to as aplasia), hypoplasia, presence of supernumerary ovaries, and atypical development, leading to the simultaneous presence of male and female gonads such as occurs in hermaphrodites. Also, normal embryonic tissue, which is not grossly evident at birth, may undergo changes in adult life, the most common of which are cystic changes of normal embryonic gonadal or ductular structures [3].

Ovarian agenesis is reported in the bitch and queen. Reports of monolateral or bilateral ovarian aplasia are anecdotal in the dog; therefore, clinical parameters for single animals are unknown. Obviously, a lack of both ovaries is likely to cause primary anestrus, however. Unlike cases in the bitch, cases of ovarian aplasia reported in the queen have always been monolateral [4–6] and, as such, unlikely to cause anestrus. Unless serial tissue sections are examined, underdeveloped gonadal tissues can easily be missed, raising the question as to whether the gonads are truly "aplastic" (not developed at all) or hypoplastic.

Ovarian hypoplasia has been reported in the bitch and queen. In the dog, it has been associated with an abnormal karyotype and with persistent anestrus or various degrees of cyclicity. In three bitches in which the results of ovarian histology were available, the ovaries were small and characterized mostly by interstitial type cells and solid epithelial sex cords, with an absence of follicles or corpora lutea. Two bitches had a 77,XO karyotype [7,8], whereas one had an X chromosomal trisomy (77,XXX) [9]. No abnormalities of the external genitalia were observed in any of these bitches. An example of ovarian hypoplasia is shown in Fig. 1.

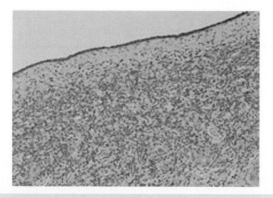

Fig. 1. The hypoplastic ovary of this 4-year-old domestic short-haired queen was small, and the surface was smooth. The photomicrograph shows the ovarian surface covered by cuboidal epithelial cells and the ovarian stroma completely devoid of oocytes, developing follicles, or other normal ovarian structures.

In the cat, bilateral ovarian hypoplasia is also a feature of abnormal chromosomal sex complement (eg, 37,XO; 37,XO/74,XXOO; 37,X/39,XXX; 37,XO/38,XX karyotypes). Queens with bilateral ovarian hypoplasia often present with primary anestrus. Four cases of cats with a 37,XO chromosome complement have been described. One was an adult female with a small uterus and small ovaries characterized histologically only by fibroblastic stromal elements and aggregates of interstitial cells [10], whereas the other three cases were kittens that died or were euthanized during the first few days of life [11–13]. Unilateral ovarian hypoplasia, also reported in the queen, may not interfere with fertility: each of two unrelated stray domestic short-haired cats that were presented for ovariohysterectomy and found to be pregnant with four and five fetuses, respectively, had one ovary that was a small 1-mm × 1-mm diameter hypoplastic nodule with no follicular structures or just small antral and preantral follicles [14].

The occurrence of supernumerary ovaries has been observed [4,15], although the histology of such accessory ovarian tissue has never been described. In a queen undergoing routine spay, two left ovaries (total of three ovaries) were found located approximately 1 cm apart on the broad ligament; their individual size was smaller that that of the right ovary, but their total mass exceeded that of the contralateral ovary [16]. Unfortunately, ovarian histology was not performed in this case, which casts doubt on the real nature of those supernumerary ovaries, because ectopic nodules of adrenal origin have been reported in many species. In the cat, they are most frequently located on the broad ligament within 1 to 4 cm from the ovary. In a survey of approximately 500 queens presented for routine ovariohysterectomy, 2.2% animals had single, bilateral, or double ipsilateral (two on the same side) paraovarian nodules [17]. Ectopic paraovarian nodules have no clinical significance. An example of ectopic adrenal tissue from a cat is shown in Fig. 2.

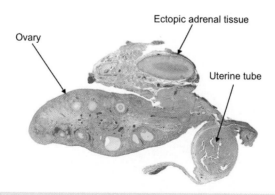

Fig. 2. Ectopic adrenal gland found adjacent to the ovary in a 2-year-old domestic short-haired queen is seen as the slightly ovoid nodule just above the ovary in this photograph. A cross section of uterine tube is present at the lower right. Although common, ectopic tissue may be small and not readily recognized grossly.

Frequently, remnants of the embryonic mesonephric (male reproductive) duct system persist into adult life in the female animal and undergo cystic distention. In queens and bitches, this is true most commonly for remnants of the mesonephric ducts and tubules. The mesonephric tubules (which develop into the rete testes in the normal male animal) form the rete ovarii in normal female animals, which may undergo cystic change in the bitch and queen. Remnants of the cranial mesonephric tubules can be found as cysts of varying size at the cranial pole of the ovary and are called cystic epoophoron (Fig. 3).

Testicular and Epididymal Abnormalities

Embryonic testicular development occurs when a gene present on the Y chromosome signals production of a testis-determining factor, which is followed by secretion of a glycoprotein hormone by the embryonic Sertoli cells called Müllerian inhibiting substance (MIS) as well as by testosterone secretion by the embryonic Leydig cells. The hormone MIS causes regressions of the Müllerian (mesonephric) duct system (which is the section of undifferentiated reproductive system giving rise in female animals to the uterine tubes, uterus, and cranial vagina) and development of the Wolffian duct system into the epididymis and vasa deferentia [1,2]. Canine testicular descent is coordinated by growth and regression of the gubernaculum (a mesenchymal structure connecting the caudal pole of the testis to the external opening of the inguinal canal) and occurs in three phases: intra-abdominal (gubernacular outgrowth and migration through the abdomen), intrainguinal (gubernacular outgrowth and migration through the inguinal canal), and extrainguinal (gubernacular regression and migration into the scrotum). Gubernacular outgrowth is mostly mediated

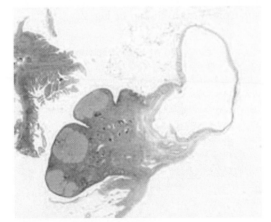

Fig. 3. The ovary of this 10-year-old mixed-breed bitch has a large cyst protruding from the cranial pole of the ovary (cystic epoophoron), which developed from a remnant piece of the mesonephric tubules. These cysts are less common than are cystic rete ovarii, which may also develop from remnants of the embryonic mesonephric tubules.

by a testicular nonandrogenic factor and only minimally by testosterone, whereas gubernacular regression is coordinated by testosterone [18]. The third phase of canine testicular descent occurs shortly after birth. According to a study done in 105 puppies, the testes start to reach the scrotum during the first week of life and both testicles are in their normal location by 42 days of age in nearly 100% of puppies [19]. Much less is known about the descent of feline testicles. Although the process of gubernacular outgrowth and regression is likely to be similar to that of the dog, the entire migration through the inguinal canal and into the scrotum occurs before birth, and feline testicles are known to move freely up and down the inguinal canal until puberty. Testicular abnormalities include the congenital absence of one (monorchidism) or both (anorchidism or aplasia) testicles, fusion of the testes into a single structure (synorchidism), presence of supernumerary testes (polyorchidism), hypoplasia of testicles (microrchidism), and presence of cystic structures within the testicular parenchyma.

Monorchidism and anorchidism
Monorchidism and anorchidism are rare conditions that may go unnoticed, because confirming their diagnosis requires a patient search at laparotomy for a blunt end of the spermatic cord(s) and testicular blood vessels; the epididymis may be found in the abdomen on the side of the missing testis [20]. Monorchidism and anorchidism as well as testicular hypoplasia have been observed in the dog [4,21,22] and the cat [4,20]. Two cases of monorchidism (in a series of 23 cryptorchid cats) and two cases of testicular aplasia (in a series of 50 cryptorchid cats) were reported in the cat [23,24]. Synorchidism and polyorchidism have never been observed in the dog or cat, although the lack of reports in the literature might mean that the problem has only escaped the attention of clinicians and pathologists to date (polyorchidism has been observed in the horse and calf [4].

Cryptorchidism and ectopia
Failure of the testicle(s) to undergo normal descent into the scrotum is defined as cryptorchidism. Failure of the testicle to complete its migration across the inguinal canal and into the scrotum is referred to as ectopia. Canine [25,26]) and feline [23,24] cryptorchidism have been reviewed. Cryptorchidism can be abdominal or inguinal, whereas ectopic testicles are typically located subcutaneously in the perineal or crural region. Incidence in the dog varies between 1% and 10% [27–29]. It is a much rarer condition in the cat (incidence less than 0.5%), although cryptorchidism is considered to be the most common congenital defect of the urogenital system in the cat [30]. The genetics of canine cryptorchidism have been well elucidated: it is a sex-linked autosomal recessive trait whose modes of inheritance and penetration are still unknown. The Toy Poodle, Pomeranian, Yorkshire Terrier, Miniature Dachshund, Cairn Terrier, Chihuahua, Maltese, Boxer, Pekingese, and English Bulldog are the first 10 breeds (in decreasing order) in a list of breeds at higher risk of cryptorchidism. Because it is an autosomal gene(s), male and female animals can both carry the trait, which means that the parents and all full siblings of the cryptorchid dog

(plus the cryptorchid animal itself) should be eliminated from the breeding line should complete removal of the cryptorchid gene pool be a priority within a canine breeding establishment. An alternative approach, such as removing only the affected dog and its parents, allows for a reduction in the trait from the population. Although genetic studies have not been done in the cat and no breeds at risk have been identified (however, Persian cats are exceedingly common in surveys of cryptorchid cats), few doubt its heritable nature and many share the view that cryptorchid tomcats should not be used as breeders. Cryptorchid dogs and cats cannot be used as show animals in official competitions.

Although not yet well defined, the pathogenesis of canine cryptorchidism has been investigated in detail over the past two decades, whereas no such study has been performed in cryptorchid cats. The presence of a strong cranial suspensory ligament has been observed in a cryptorchid dog, the failure of which to break down has been supposed to prevent gubernacular outgrowth and migration [31]. An increased risk of cryptorchidism has been identified in smaller individuals within a given breed [32]. No difference in basal serum estrogen concentrations and inconsistent differences in basal serum luteinizing hormone (LH) or testosterone concentrations (occasionally lower in cryptorchid animals) have been observed between normal and cryptorchid dogs [33,34], whereas post–gonadotropin-releasing hormone (GnRH) serum testosterone is lower in cryptorchid dogs than in normal dogs [35]. The use of GnRH has been anecdotally reported as helping testicular descent in cryptorchid dogs, but its success has not been consistent. Failure to identify a single cause or an ideal treatment probably indicates that the condition is multifactorial, with physical as well as endocrine factors contributing to preventing gubernacular outgrowth or regression or making testicular size incompatible with the size of the inguinal canal.

Cryptorchidism in the dog and cat is definitively diagnosed at puberty, because closure of the inguinal rings is complete at that time, which makes further movement of retained testicles impossible. Movements of testicles up and down the inguinal canal before its closure is much more common in cats than in dogs, which explains why approximately 25% of testicles diagnosed as cryptorchid before 6 months of age have reached the scrotum in puppies [19], although this percentage is perceived to be much higher in kittens [36]. Transit through the inguinal canal is probably also a reflection of testicular diameter: therefore, animals of precocious breeds (eg, small-sized or mongrel dogs) in which testicular growth progresses more rapidly may be confirmed at a younger age than large- or giant-sized dogs maturing later in life. In general, it is advisable to wait until 6 months of age before confirming the diagnosis of cryptorchidism [37]. Because the number of genes involved as well as their penetrance is unknown, one should wonder whether testicular descent after 45 days of age in the dog (and after birth in the cat) should be considered a potential indication of abnormality, at least of the inguinal canal (if not of the testicle itself), which might put offspring at a higher risk of developing the condition.

In cryptorchid testicles, hormonal production is variably affected but generally maintained, whereas sperm production is absent regardless of abdominal or inguinal location. In cats, male phenotype and behavior, libido, aggressiveness, and tomcat urine odor are maintained in unilateral cryptorchid male animals after removal of the scrotal testicle; all such features disappear after removal of the cryptorchid testicle [38–40]. Bilaterally cryptorchid dogs and cats are generally azoospermic, and dogs with such a condition have been shown to be unable to achieve an erection [41], whereas unilateral cryptorchid male animals may have a slightly lower fertility but should be considered potentially sound as breeders [28]. Apart from a slightly lower fertility, unilaterally cryptorchid dogs and cats are clinically normal, although the presence of a few congenital defects has been reported, such as patellar luxation (in dogs and cats); a shortened or kinked tail; tarsal deformity; tetralogy of Fallot; microphthalmia or upper eyelid agenesis (in cats) [24]; and inguinal hernia, umbilical hernia, hip dysplasia, and penile or preputial defects (in dogs) [32,42].

The abdominal and inguinal locations are also characterized by an increased incidence of testicular tumors in affected dogs, perhaps because of the higher temperature of the abdominal or inguinal cavity. The risk of developing neoplasia in a retained (abdominal or inguinal) canine testicle is 9 to 13 times higher than in a scrotal testicle [32,42], with Sertoli cell tumor and seminoma being the most common types of neoplasia developing in retained testicles. The increased testicular size (and the fact that abdominal testicles are loosely suspended from the abdominal vault) increases the possibility of torsion of the spermatic cord, a likely outcome of abdominal retention in adult dogs [43–47]. The high risk of developing testicular neoplasia as well as the risk of developing bone marrow hypoplasia (with leukopenia and thrombocytopenia) in dogs with a feminizing syndrome caused by a Sertoli cell tumor makes removal of cryptorchid testicles imperative and bilateral castration highly recommended (to decrease possible transmission of a hereditary defect) in the dog. Removal of ectopic testes is advised also on general (rather than just reproductive) health grounds because they are more exposed to chronic trauma as a result of their location. In cats, torsion of the spermatic cord has never been reported, and testicular tumors are rare and not found in cryptorchid cats, although surgery is typically performed in young animals [38].

HERMAPHRODITISM

An abnormality of chromosomal, gonadal, or phenotypic sex leads to the contemporaneous presence of male and female internal or external genitalia or to the presence of ambiguous or hypoplastic external genitalia. The fact that the gender of individuals with such an abnormality is not clearly evident leads to generically referring to these patients as hermaphrodites or intersex. Although generic, such terms help to convey to our clients the message that their pets may have some serious (perhaps hereditary) problem affecting their reproductive system. However, it is important to realize that a large variety of potential underlying conditions are implied by the terms *intersex* or *hermaphrodite*.

The contemporaneous presence of ovarian and testicular tissue characterizes a true hermaphrodite, which is a rare condition typically characterized by histologic evidence of ovarian and testicular tissues on the same gonad, defined as an ovotestis (Fig. 4). True hermaphrodites can also have an ovary on one side and a testicle on the opposite side, which is defined as lateral hermaphroditism. True hermaphrodites can be the result of an abnormality of chromosomal sex (chimera) or an abnormality of gonadal sex (XX male animal).

As opposed to true hermaphroditism, pseudohermaphroditism is an abnormality of phenotypic sex, which refers to presence of gonads of one sex and external genitalia of the opposite sex. This is a relatively more common condition, which is defined according to the gender of the gonad: a male pseudohermaphrodite has testicles and a female phenotype, whereas a female pseudohermaphrodite has ovaries and a male phenotype. True hermaphrodites as well as pseudohermaphrodites have been repeatedly described in small animals. Although true hermaphroditism in cats is relatively rare (only true hermaphrodite chimeras have been reported), canine true hermaphroditism and related abnormalities have been recorded, particularly in Cocker Spaniels, Miniature Schnauzers, and Beagles. Table 1 features a comprehensive subdivision of all reproductive abnormalities of dogs and cats depending on whether the problem is at the level of chromosomal, gonadal, or phenotypic sex.

Abnormalities of Chromosomal Sex

These conditions can be caused by (1) nondisjunction of a sex chromosome during meiosis, leading to a gamete containing an XXY, XO, or XXX sex chromosome complement; (2) fusion of two zygotes differing in sex chromosome constitution, leading to a chimera (eg, XX/XY); or (3) fusion of cell populations with different chromosome constitutions originating within the same individual, leading to a mosaic. The XXY syndrome gives rise to a phenotypic male with hypoplastic testicles without spermatogenesis. This condition

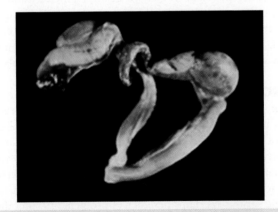

Fig. 4. Internal organs of a true hermaphrodite bitch. The gonads at the apex of the uterine horns are mostly testicular, but ovarian tissues were present. A prominent epididymis is adjacent to the ovotestis on the left. Further comments on the clinical significance of an ovotestis are provided in the legend for Fig. 5.

(Klinefelter's syndrome in human beings) occurs in dogs and is particularly well known in cats [48–51] because of the fact that tomcats with this condition often feature a calico or tortoiseshell coat. In cats, the genes for orange and nonorange coat color are alleles of the X-linked orange locus. The presence of just one allele gives rise to the orange or nonorange (black or chocolate brown) color, which is what occurs in normal male cats, whereas the tortoiseshell pattern can occur only in female cats because of heterozygosity for this allele producing patches of different hair color. Therefore, male cats with this coat color pattern must have two X chromosomes (XXY male), although a chimera or mosaic sex chromosome constitution may also produce the calico pattern. The XXY syndrome is also reported in dogs, although it is not as easy to identify because no coat color paradox exists in this species.

The XO syndrome (Turner's syndrome in human beings) is characterized by individuals that develop as phenotypic female animals with infantile genitalia; a few somatic abnormalities, including short stature; and, notably, an absence of ovaries or ovarian hypoplasia. This condition as well as the XXX chromosome constitution is reported in dogs and cats (see section on ovarian abnormalities).

When two zygotes with different sex chromosome constitutions fuse, an XX/XY individual originates, whereas when fusion occurs between two or more cell populations originating from the same individual but with different chromosome constitutions, a mosaic is produced. In these individuals, gonadal sex depends on the distribution of XX or XY cells within the gonadal ridge. The presence of an XX cell population gives rise to ovarian tissue, the presence of an XY cell population gives rise to testicular tissue, and the various degrees of their mixture produce different varieties of ovotestis or an individual with one ovary and one testicle. The presence of an ovotestis or of an ovary and a testicle defines the individual as a true hermaphrodite—in this case, a true hermaphrodite chimera. In true hermaphrodite chimeras, if a significant proportion of the XY cell population is present, the individual can be a fertile male animal, whereas if a significant proportion of cells have an XXY chromosomal pattern, the phenotype is similar to that of the XXY syndrome. Chimeras with XX/XY and XY/XY cell populations have been described in dogs and cats. A female Old English Sheepdog with primary anestrus by 2 years of age had an XX/XY cell ratio of approximately 1:1, a vulva-like structure with a hypoplastic penis, no scrotum, small retained testicles, and a hypoplastic uterus. Several cats with a chimeric XX/XY cell distribution have been reported as male animals with small to normal scrotal testicle(s), variable fertility, the presence or absence of Müllerian duct organs, and a ratio between normal and aspermic seminiferous tubules corresponding to the ratio between XX and XY cells within the testis [48,49,52].

With regard to the tortoiseshell pattern, in addition to having an XXY syndrome, male cats with this coat color may be XX/XY chimeras [52] or XY/XY chimeras [53]. In that case, normal testicular histology and normal spermatogenesis may be present.

Table 1
Abnormalities of the reproductive system in dogs and cats

	Abnormalities of chromosomal sex	Abnormalities of gonadal sex	Abnormalities of phenotypic sex
Main feature(s)	Underdeveloped genitalia; phenotype (male or female) is not ambiguous	Chromosomal and gonadal sex are not in agreement; external genitalia can be normal, abnormal or ambiguous	Internal and external genitalia are not in agreement; external genitalia can be normal, abnormal, or ambiguous
Condition(s) identified	XXY, XO, and XXX syndrome's; chimeras and mosaics (TH chimeras, XX/XY or XY/XY chimeras)	XX sex reversal, divided into: XX TH, (with at least one ovotestis) XX male (with bilateral testes)	FP: female karyotype and reproductive tract, male phenotype. MP: male karyotype, female phenotype
Reported in	DSH cats (XXY), one crossbred dog (XXY), Dobermann Pinscher (XO), Burmese and DHS cats (XO)	English Cocker Spaniel, Beagle, Weimaraner, Kerry Blue Terrier, Chinese Pug, German ShortHaired Pointer, Soft-Coated Wheaton terrier, Pomeranian, Dobermann Pinscher; not observed in cats	FP: Greyhound, Pekingese × Poodle cross, crossbred Collie: not observed in cats MP: Miniature Schnauzer, Basset Hound, Persian cat, DSH cat
Etiology	Nondisjunction of sex chromosomes during meiosis	Autosomal recessive trait (in American Cocker Spaniels)	FP: iatrogenic because of steroid administration around mid-pregnancy (day 34–36 after LH) MP: PMD is an autosomal recessive trait Hypospadia can be caused by teratogenic drugs but is also a familial defect in the dog TF is an X-linked recessive trait
Clinical features	XXY: phenotypic male with small testicles devoid of spermatozoa (cat: tortoiseshell or calico male) XO and XXX: phenotypic female with primary anestrus Chimeras: from normal male or female animal to any possible degree of abnormality, depending on amount and distribution of normal (XX, XY) cell populations	XX TH: from normal female external genitalia to severe clitoral enlargement (with os clitoris) XX male: male phenotype with male abnormal external genitalia (caudally displaced prepuce, hypospadia, and bilateral cryptorchidism) and a uterus	FP: male animals with periodic signs of estrus, attractiveness to other animals, pyometra, urinary incontinence MP: PMD: XY male animals with bilateral discended or cryptorchid testes, male internal genitalia but also female internal genitalia Hypospadia: normal male with urethral opening ventral or caudal to the penis

Is fertility possible?	No, except for chimeras with a significant proportion of XY or XX cell populations	No, except for some XX TH's that may occasionally cycle and conceive	TF: XY male animals with bilateral testes, a bifid scrotum, female phenotype, sometimes ambiguous genitalia FP: no MP: PMD: yes; Hypospadia: yes; TF: no
Diagnosis	Karyotype (in some cases, such as with tortoiseshell male cats, a karyotype may not be necessary)	Confirmation of karyotype 78,XX and presence of at least one testis or ovotestis (testosterone stimulation test)	FP: Karyotype, testosterone stimulation test (to rule out XX male) and ovarian histology MP: PMD: karyotype, bilateral testes, and presence of all Mullerian duct organs TF: karyotype, bilateral testes, and positive testosterone-stimulating test Hypospadia: clinical observation
Genetic counseling	Siblings and parents of affected individuals are healthy (it is a chance event)	Familial disorder: both parents and at least two third of male and female siblings of affected individuals are carriers	FP: siblings and parents of affected individuals are healthy Hypospadia: being a familial disorder, it is better to avoid breeding affected individuals PMD and TF: do not breed affected and carrier individuals; carrier female animals are fertile, and 50% of their male offspring are affected, whereas 50% of their female offspring are carriers

The most common congenital disfunctions of canine and feline reproductive organs are classified according to where in the reproductive devepment process (chromosomal, gonadal, or phenotypic sex) the problem originates. This table is intended to help readers establish a connection between a clinical sign and the underlying disease, thus loccating quickly the section of this article where the related information may befound.

Abbreviations: DSH, domestic short-haired; TF, testicular feminization; FP, female pseudohermaphrodite; LH, luteinizing hormone; MP, male pseudohermaphrodite; PMD, persistence of Müllerian ducts; TH, true hermaphrodite.

Abnormalities of Gonadal Sex

When gonadal sex develops in an abnormal way, its end product, be it ovary or testicle, disagrees with the sex chromosome complement of the individual. This condition is called sex reversed and theoretically gives rise to XX male and XY female animals. Whereas XY sex reversal has been described in other mammals, only XX sex reversal is reported in dogs, particularly in English Cocker Spaniels, Beagles, Weimaraners, Kerry Blue Terriers, Chinese Pugs, German Short-Haired Pointers, Soft-Coated Wheaton Terriers, Pomeranians, and Doberman Pinschers [1,2,54–56]. Depending on the degree of testicular tissue development, an ovotestis, both gonads, an ovotestis and a gonad (XX true hermaphrodite), or testicles only (XX male syndrome) may be present. The sex-reversed condition has not been observed in cats.

XX true hermaphrodite

In addition to the contemporaneous presence of both gonads, these hermaphrodites often have portions of the reproductive tracts and external genitalia belonging to both sexes, although their phenotype is most commonly female. An ovary can be present on one side and a testicle on the other side (described as lateral hermaphroditism), or ovarian and testicular tissues can be present on the same gonad (ovotestis) (see Fig. 5).

The presence of an ovotestis is generally characterized by one or more abnormalities of the reproductive system, although the tubular tract may be normal in XX true hermaphrodite bitches, which often complicates the diagnostic process. For instance, Selden and colleagues [57] described a case of a true hermaphrodite bitch with a normal 78,XX karyotype that reproduced. In

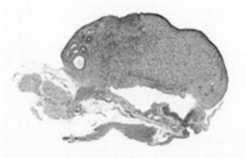

Fig. 5. The cellular features of this ovotestis taken from a true hermaphrodite bitch are evident in this subgross photograph of a midlongitudinal section of the gonad. Most of the gonad contains lobules of hypoplastic seminiferous tubules, but ovarian tissue containing several variably sized follicles is clearly evident at the left pole. Unless karyotyping is performed, it is not possible to distinguish whether this is a chromosomal (chimera) or gonadal (XX male) sex abnormality. Such a distinction is useful in clinical practice for genetic counseling, because siblings of XX male individuals may carry the trait and may spread the defect across the population, whereas this does not occur for chimeras.

addition, a case of lateral hermaphroditism has been described in a phenotypically normal female Weimaraner that had a normal female karyotype, normal tubular reproductive tract, and occurrence of irregular oestrus cycles [118]. Cases of bilateral ovotestis have been described in two Cocker Spaniels, a German Short-Haired Pointer, and a mongrel dog; these dogs had a normal female phenotype and karyotype (78,XX), normal female tubular reproductive tract, and an enlarged clitoris with an os penis [58–61].

XX true hermaphroditism is rarely observed in tomcats and is never reported in queens. An ovotestis with an oviduct and uterine horn entering the urethra (all structures were on the right side of the abdomen) was found in a male cat on necropsy; the cat had a normal penis and prostate and a scrotal testicle on the left side of the scrotum [62]. A 4-year-old American short-haired tomcat presented for long-lasting urinary incontinence and hematuria was reported to have bilateral ovotestes and a thin-walled uterus. Surgical removal of the uterus and gonads corrected the urologic problem [63].

XX Male Syndrome
The major characteristic of XX male animals is the presence of bilateral, often cryptorchid, testes. Clinical features of this condition also include a caudally displaced prepuce and penile malformations, such as hypospadia, hypoplasia, or abnormal curvature. The presence of only some sections of the female reproductive system (uterus) but not others (oviduct) implies a lack of sensitivity of target organs to MIS.

Diagnosis of the XX sex-reversed condition requires a karyotype and histologic confirmation of at least one ovotestis or testis. A testosterone stimulation test may help, although a lack of testosterone elevation after administration of GnRH or human chorionic gonadotropin (hCG) may not rule out the presence of an XX sex-reversed condition. XX male animals are always sterile and should undergo removal of cryptorchid testicles and a uterus as soon as diagnosed, whereas some XX true hermaphrodites may show estrous cycles and occasionally produce offspring [56]. Breeding affected dogs should be strongly discouraged, however, because affected individuals are homozygous for the (autosomal recessive) sex-reversed trait and their offspring are affected or are carriers of the malformation. Furthermore, because this is a homozygous gene, parents of affected dogs are obviously carriers, as are at least two thirds of male and female siblings.

Abnormalities of Phenotypic Sex
Individuals with ambiguity of internal or external genitalia are defined as being pseudohermaphrodites. Male pseudohermaphrodites are female-looking individuals with a normal male karyotype, whereas female pseudohermaphrodites have a female karyotype and a male phenotype.

Female Pseudohermaphroditism
These individuals have an XX karyotype, a female tubular reproductive tract, ovaries, and a male phenotype with a penis and prepuce. This condition occurs

rarely in all species and is often the result of masculinization of female fetuses because of exposure to exogenous steroids in utero, such as treating the mother with androgens or progestogens before or during pregnancy [59,64–66]. The incidence of female pseudohermaphroditism might be underestimated because of the fact that dogs with this condition may rarely show cyclic activity of their internal female reproductive system, and are therefore unlikely to be referred to the veterinarian for reproductive reasons unless the owner wants to use them for breeding purposes. Urovagina (urinary stasis in the proximal vagina) and urinary incontinence have been reported in female pseudohermaphrodites: a 1-year-old Pekingese-Poodle cross female pseudohermaphrodite had experienced urinary incontinence for 5 months, which improved after an ovariohysterectomy; however, the dog subsequently developed estrogen-responsive urinary incontinence [65]. Diagnosis requires karyotyping and histologic confirmation of the presence of ovaries. Also, ruling out the presence of an XX sex-reversed condition (using a testosterone stimulation test) may be important for genetic counseling; although female pseudohermaphroditism has no genetic implication, parents and siblings of XX true hermaphrodites are carriers of the trait and should be removed from the breeding stock. Gonadal histology is fundamental in case no testosterone production is observed. Therefore, female pseudohermaphrodites should undergo an ovariectomy, and the ovaries should be submitted for histologic examination. Because of the risk of urinary tract malformations (some of which may require surgery), contrast studies of the posterior urogenital tract are indicated in these animals before an ovariectomy. To reduce the incidence of these problems, it is best to avoid steroid administration during pregnancy, particularly during gestational days 34 to 46 after the administration of LH, which is when the development of canine and feline internal and external genitalia takes place [67,68].

Male Pseudohermaphroditism
Male pseudohermaphrodites are female-looking individuals with a normal male karyotype, retained testes, a uterus masculinus, and a vulva that may show an enlarged clitoris [69]. This condition can be caused by failure of the Müllerian duct to regress or failure of androgens to effect masculinization of target organs.

Persistence of Müllerian ducts
Failure of Müllerian ducts to regress is probably attributable to the absence of MIS receptors, because MIS is regularly produced during the embryonic critical period in animals with this condition [56]. The result is the development of the Wolffian (male reproductive) and Müllerian (female reproductive) organs in the same individual. Affected animals have an XY karyotype with bilateral testes (cryptorchid in approximately 50% of the cases) and a normal male reproductive system but also bilateral oviducts, a complete uterus with a cervix, and a cranial vagina. Being normal male animals by all means, these individuals may go unnoticed until they develop pyometra or a urinary tract or prostatic infection. This condition has been widely documented in Miniature

Schnauzers in the United States and in Basset Hounds in The Netherlands, and it has also been observed in Persian cats [1,2].

A male pseudohermaphrodite 1-year-old blue tabby queen was reported to have abdominal testes at the tip of the uterine horns and remnants of the Müllerian duct system [70]). Although a karyotype was not identified, no Barr bodies (sex chromatin) were found on 400 cells from the oral mucosa, indicating the lack of a normal XX chromosome complement. Signs of estrus have been observed in phenotypically male cats with a small penis visible through the vulvar labia, ovaries, and uterus [71,72]. Although this might be considered indicative of pseudohermaphroditism, no results of ovarian histology was available, which does not rule out the presence of an ovotestis, because the penis does not develop without androgen stimulation. A previously castrated 6-year-old domestic long-haired tomcat with a 38,XY karyotype, which was referred for persistent dysuria, was found to have a uterus masculinus; dysuria had developed after a perineal urethrostomy performed 2 weeks earlier, and the uterus was compressing the urethral lumen at the level of the trigone [73]. In another young, neutered male cat pyometra of the uterus masculinus was reported to cause stranguria, lethargy, and antibiotic-responsive fever [117]. In both cases clinical signs resolved following hysterectomy [73,117].

Diagnosis of the persistence of Müllerian ducts is based on karyotype and the presence of bilateral testes as well as that of all Müllerian duct organs. Castration and hysterectomy are the treatment of choice. When removing the uterus, it is important to remove as much vagina as possible, because small-diameter communications between the cranial vagina and prostatic urethra (which may be a source of ascending infection to the uterus) have been observed [56]. As for genetic counseling, persistence of Müllerian ducts is attributable to an autosomal recessive gene, which means that only homozygous male animals express the phenotype. Parents and males and females siblings of affected individuals can be carriers and should be eliminated from the breeding stock.

Defects in androgen-dependent masculinization

For male genitalia and secondary sex characteristics to develop normally, three conditions must be satisfied: testosterone secretion, its conversion to dihydrotestosterone (DHT) in target organs, and the presence of androgen receptors at the target organs. A defect in any of these three steps causes partial or total failure of masculinization. Although no defect in androgen production or in conversion from testosterone to DHT has been reported in dogs and cats, a specific androgen receptor defect observed in both species is testicular feminization, a congenital and hereditary syndrome. Minor conditions that may be attributable to incomplete masculinization include hypospadia and persistence of the penile frenulum (see section on abnormalities of the penis and prepuce), although the former can be also caused by teratogens. Also, cryptorchidism has been proposed as being caused by a defect in androgen-dependent masculinization [2,56]. However, the potential role of failure of masculinization in the underlying mechanism of cryptorchidism has not been established yet.

Testicular feminization is characterized by the presence of normal testes that secrete testosterone but no androgen receptors in target tissues; although androgens inhibit development of the female internal genitalia, absence of their receptors inhibits development of the whole male excurrent tract. Such a syndrome has been observed in a dog and in a few cats. A mixed-breed XY male dog with bilateral testes in a bifid scrotum had normal peripheral concentrations of testosterone and DHT after stimulation with hCG (see section on diagnostic and clinical approach) as well as the presence of testosterone receptors but an absence of DHT receptors in cultured genital fibroblasts [74]. The presence of both epididymides in this dog may be explained by the selective action of testosterone stimulating growth and differentiation of some parts of the Wolffian duct system during embryonic development. A lack of DHT receptors is bound to impair pubertal growth and proper functioning of the male reproductive system. A 6-month-old orange tabby queen with a 38,XY chromosome complement had abdominal testes, a normal vulva, and the complete absence of uterus, oviducts (as expected, because MIS production was normal), as well as the absence of the epididymis and vasa deferentia, and no androgen receptors were found in cultured fibroblasts taken from the genital skin [75]. Dogs and cats with this problem should undergo a gonadectomy (performed in human beings with this syndrome because of the risk of testicular neoplasia), followed by gonadal histologic evaluation to confirm the diagnosis [1,2].

ABNORMALITIES OF THE FEMALE TUBULAR GENITAL TRACT
Uterus, Uterine Tube, and Cervical Abnormalities

The absence of secretion of MIS (secreted by the embryonic testis) in the female fetus allows full development of the Müllerian duct system, which gives rise to the uterine tubes, uterus, and cranial vagina [1,2].

Congenital anomalies reported in the canine uterus and uterine tubes include unilateral aplasia (also termed *uterus unicornis*), partial fusion, and unequal development of one of the two uterine horns. Unilateral uterine aplasia has been reported in dogs and cats [76–78]. When one uterine horn is absent, the ovary and uterine tube are generally present on the affected side [76]. The ovaries and oviducts derive from a different embryologic origin, the gonadal ridge, whereas the rest of the female tubular tract derives from the paramesonephric ducts and urogenital sinus. When an abnormality of one uterine horn is observed, one should always consider the possibility of other abnormalities being present at the affected site; for instance, uterus unicornis and agenesis of the ipsilateral kidney have been observed in female cats [5,79]. Partial or complete fusion or occlusion of one uterine horn (segmental aplasia) may also cause fluid accumulation in that horn or in the entire uterus, depending on the level at which the occlusion is located. Such unilateral problems are often observed only on routine ovariohysterectomy, because the presence of normal reproductive structures on just one side may allow the female animal to cycle and conceive without any apparent remarkable deviation from normality (although a small litter size may be observed). Fig. 6 shows a case of feline unilateral

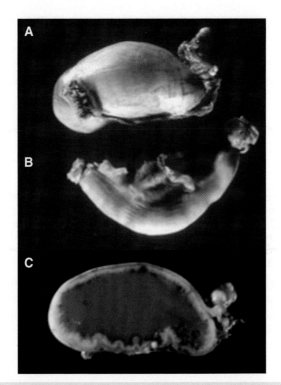

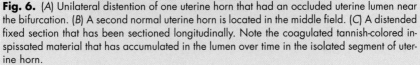

Fig. 6. (A) Unilateral distention of one uterine horn that had an occluded uterine lumen near the bifurcation. (B) A second normal uterine horn is located in the middle field. (C) A distended fixed section that has been sectioned longitudinally. Note the coagulated tannish-colored inspissated material that has accumulated in the lumen over time in the isolated segment of uterine horn.

segmental stenosis with distention of the proximal segment of the affected uterine horn.

Mesonephric duct remnants are less commonly found in dogs and cats than in large domestic animals. Occasionally, cysts or short distended tubular segments derived from persisting embryonic remnants of the mesonephric ducts are found along the uterine tubes or along the uterine horn on the mesometrial attachment (Fig. 7). These are considered incidental findings because they generally bear little if any clinical relevance.

Abnormalities of the uterus and uterine tubes are common in intersex animals, particularly in male pseudohermaphrodites and true hermaphrodites [80]. Male pseudohermaphrodites may have the so-called "uterus masculinus" (a remnant of the paramesonephric duct) or normal uterine horns, which are blind-ended, suggesting an abnormality of the uterine tubes. Lateral true hermaphrodites may have an abnormal uterus or uterine tube on the side of the testicle [37]. Female pseudohermaphrodites as well as sex-reversed animals

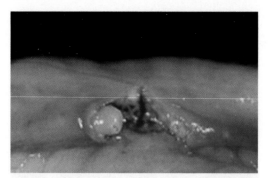

Fig. 7. The uterine horn of this otherwise normal 5-year-old bitch had a small (approximately 5 mm in diameter) cystic mesonephric duct remnant adjacent to the uterine horn. These are invariably located on the side of attachment of the broad ligament and are not associated with any effects on fertility.

are reported to have normal uteri [59,69,81]. Careful examination of the uterine walls of intersex bitches may reveal remnants of the male mesonephric duct (Fig. 8). Bilateral blockage of uterine tubes due to villous or papillary hyperplasia is reported in queens as a cause of infertility [80,116].

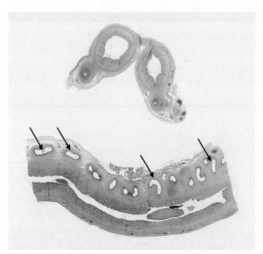

Fig. 8. Subgross photograph of uterine tissue taken from an intersex dog shows uterine- and vas-like structures (derived from paramesonephric and mesonephric embryonic ducts, respectively). In the upper cross section of the horns near their bifurcation, the cross section of two smaller ducts, lined by cuboidal epithelium, is present near the attachment of the broad ligaments. These are paired mesonephric ducts, which would be the vas deferens in a normal male dog. The tissue at the bottom of the photograph shows a longitudinal section of one uterine horn with the mesonephric duct running in and out of the plane of section (several oblique sections of the duct are labeled with *arrows*).

Agenesis of the cervix has been reported in a bitch with the uterine body ending blindly; the uterus was separated from the vagina by membranous tissue, thus becoming distended with fluid [82].

ABNORMALITIES OF THE MALE EXCURRENT TRACT AND ACCESSORY SEX GLANDS

Epididymis, Deferens, and Prostate Abnormalities

The excurrent tract includes the rete testis, efferent ducts, epididymis, vas deferens, and urethra. The accessory glands of small animals are the prostate and ampullae of the deferens (dog) and the prostate and bulbourethral (or Cowper's) gland (tomcat). Complete or partial absence of the epididymis may occur, albeit rarely, in the dog [4]. The canine epididymis has also been observed to be increased or decreased in size, with single or multiple occlusions of its duct, as well as being abnormally located within the scrotum [4]. Congenital epididymal or bulbourethral abnormalities have never been observed in the cat.

Prostatic hypoplasia

Congenital prostatic hypoplasia or aplasia is rare in the dog and cat and is usually associated with developmental anomalies, such as hermaphroditism or pseudohermaphroditism. Hypoplasia is generally the result of the absence of testosterone from the general circulation. Being an accessory sex gland, the prostate needs an adequate androgen concentration to grow and start functioning. Prostatic hypoplasia caused by endocrine insufficiency can therefore only be detected after puberty, although hypoandrogenism becomes noticeable because of signs other than prostatic hypoplasia (eg, lack of libido, insufficient body growth, puppy behavior). The dorsal longitudinal median groove dividing the prostate in two halves is occasionally absent in the dog, which may erroneously be perceived as a sign of prostatic hypertrophy in a young animal. Prostatic hypertrophy cannot develop without the presence of testosterone or its active metabolite, DHT, in the general circulation. Therefore, the observation of a larger than normal prostate in a young animal can only be attributed to precocious puberty or a testosterone-producing tumor.

Cystic rete testis

A case of cystic rete testis was observed in an 8-month-old cat at routine castration [83]. The cystic structure occupied approximately half of the right testis and was communicating with a smaller cyst in the head of the right epididymis. Areas of active spermatogenesis alternated with areas of focal degeneration in the right testis, whereas no sperm was present in the right epididymis. No such alteration has been reported yet in the dog.

ABNORMALITIES OF EXTERNAL GENITALIA

Abnormalities of the Vagina, Vestibule, and Vulva

The uterus, cervix, cranial vagina, and vestibule develop from the paired Müllerian ducts (or paramesonephric ducts), which fuse during embryonic life. A papillary projection of the caudal tip of each of these ducts pushes forward into the urogenital sinus to form the Müllerian tubercle, which becomes canalized and fuses to the genital fold, forming the vestibule. The vulvar lips develop from the genital swellings, and the clitoris originates from the genital tubercle. The hymen develops at the junction between the Müllerian ducts and the urogenital sinus, and it is usually open at birth in dogs and cats [84]. An incomplete fusion of each of these three embryonic structures within themselves and with each other causes developmental problems at specific sites of the reproductive system (Table 2).

Vaginal septa, an imperforate hymen, vaginovestibular strictures, vestibulovulvar strictures, segmental aplasia of the vagina, and vulvar agenesis have been described in the bitch [85–90], whereas only an imperforate hymen has been observed in the queen [91]. The most commonly reported vaginal anomalies of the dog are vaginal septa and circumferential vaginovestibular strictures. Although the reported incidence is low (0.003%) [89], the true incidence could be higher, because many cases probably go unnoticed if the bitch is not used for breeding. Signs of vaginal septa or strictures may be absent or may include vaginitis, inability to breed naturally, urinary incontinence (most common) or urinary tract infections, dystocia, infertility, and ambiguous external genitalia (less common). A vaginal stricture in a Beagle bitch is shown in Fig. 9.

Clitoral hypertrophy is also reported as a congenital problem in the bitch, which can be caused by treating the dam with progestogens or androgens during pregnancy or by the presence of functional testicular tissue in case of abnormalities of gonadal or phenotypic sex (Figs. 10 and 11) [69]. Clitoral hypertrophy was reported in 52% of 25 male pseudohermaphrodite dogs and in 100% of 13 true hermaphrodite dogs [69]. In intersex individuals, the clitoris generally starts growing at puberty when testicular secretion begins to increase. Clitoral hypertrophy frequently persists even once the cause has been removed, which often makes clitoridectomy a necessary treatment.

Congenital abnormalities of feline external genitalia include segmental aplasia of the cranial vagina, an impatent vagina and persistent hymen, the presence of a common vulvovestibular-anal opening, and a rectovaginal fistula [4,91]. In nonbreeding animals, abnormalities of the cranial vagina may go unnoticed or may cause the uterus to become fluid filled, whereas they may cause failure to

Table 2
Relation between developmental defects attributable to incomplete fusion of the embryonic undifferentiated reproductive organs (Müllerian duct system) and related anomaly of the female reproductive tract in dogs and cats

Incomplete fusion	Causes
Müllerian ducts with themselves	Vertical vaginal septa or double vagina
Müllerian ducts and urogenital sinus	Incomplete perforation of the hymen
Genital swellings and genital folds	Vestibulovulvar strictures or hypoplasia

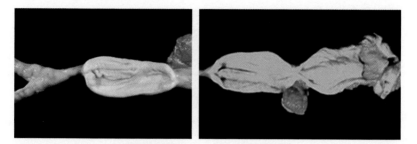

Fig. 9. The cranial half of the vagina of this Beagle bitch was distended with tan slightly viscous fluid. (*Left panel*) Opened distended segment extends from the cervix (external os is visible at the left end of the vaginal lumen) to the area of vaginal stenosis at the right end of the opened segment. (*Right panel*) The entire vagina and vulva with an area of stenosis in the middle segment of the vagina, proximal to the urethra orifice, is shown. The round structure extending below the middle section of the vagina in the area of the stricture is the bladder.

conceive in breeding queens. In adult queens, an impatent vagina might be a consequence of previous dystocia. Vulvovestibular anomalies can be observed by careful inspection of external genitalia in kittens and puppies and can often be corrected surgically.

Abnormalities of the Penis and Prepuce

Canine and feline male external genitalia originate from the urogenital tubercle (which forms at the level of the embryonic cloacal membrane) around day 25 after conception as a direct result of the influence of DHT (converted from testosterone by the enzyme 5-a-reductase). The prepuce develops from a circular plate of ectoderm invaginating at the level of the distal tip of the penis, whereas the junction between the preputial and penile mucosa (balanopreputial fold) dissolves at a later stage thanks to the action of androgens [92]. The most

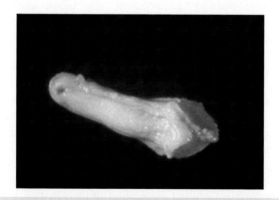

Fig. 10. An enlarged clitoris, approximately 3 cm in length, protruded from between the vulvar lips of an intersex (true hermaphrodite) bitch. An os clitoris was present. Only rarely does the clitoris of normal bitches contain bone (os clitoris).

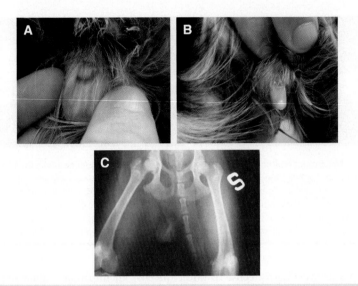

Fig. 11. Clitoral hypertrophy in a 6-month-old English Cocker Spaniel. An enlarged clitoris can be noted dilating the vulvar lips (A) and can be fully appreciated in its dimensions on exterioration by applying forward pressure against each vulvar lip (B). (C) On a ventrodorsal radiographic study, ossification of the os clitoris can be observed. Such a malformation can be caused by an abnormality of gonadal or phenotypic sex (see Table 1). Once such a degree of hypertrophy is attained, the clitoris does not generally decrease in size, even after removing the source of endogenous or exogenous androgens. Its presence is often responsible for chronic vaginal inflammation, and clitoridectomy is required.

common congenital abnormalities of the penis and prepuce in dogs and cats are duplication of the penis (diphallia), failure of the balanopreputial fold to separate (penile frenulum), termination of the penile urethra at an abnormal location (hypospadia), inability to protrude the penis from the prepuce (phimosis), preputial hypoplasia, penile immaturity, and penile hypoplasia. With the exception of diphallia, all other abnormalities may be observed in intersex animals.

A duplication of the cloacal membrane early in the course of embryonic development may lead to duplication of the urogenital tubercle, causing duplication of the penis, which is referred to as diphallia, a congenital problem that has been reported in three 5- to 6-month-old dogs: a Pointer, a Poodle, and a mixed-breed dog [3,93,94]. All three dogs were presented for urinary tract signs (hematuria, pollakiuria, and inappropriate urination) and also showed complete duplication of the urinary bladder. A chromosomal analysis performed in two dogs revealed a normal karyotype (78,XY). Other features of this congenital problem included duplication of the prostate, a bifid scrotum, bilateral cryptorchidism, renal hypoplasia, and bifurcation of the descending colon. Dogs with diphallia may live a normal life, although urinary tract infections tend to recur. Kidney status and function need to be evaluated closely, especially if monolateral renal hypoplasia is present. In one case, the affected dog was euthanized because of right renal hypoplasia and pyelonephritis of the other kidney [95]. Although causes of duplication of the cloacal membrane are currently unknown, diphallia is thought to be a chance event and, as such, should be self-limiting; therefore, it is probably wise to avoid breeding a dog with such a problem, but it is probably safe to breed the parents and siblings of affected individuals.

The frenulum is a thin membrane of connective tissue joining the ventral aspect of the tip of the penis to the prepuce or the corpus of the penis. Its presence is attributable to the fact that dissolution of the balanopreputial fold (an androgen-dependent process) did not occur normally. Persistence of the penile frenulum has been reported in 24 dogs, most of which were Cocker Spaniels (almost all from the same kennel) and 4 of which were Poodles [96–100]. Persistence of the penile frenulum has been observed in tomcats (Fig. 12). Presenting complaints include excessive licking, dermatitis between the rear limbs caused by urine dribbling, curvature of the penis during erection (or phallocampsis), pain at breeding, and low libido. Some dogs, especially if never used as studs, may be fully asymptomatic, which explains the wide age range at first diagnosis of 3 months to 8 years [96–100]. A persistent frenulum can be transected under a light plane of general anesthesia or even local anesthesia (thin frenula may be snipped with scissors without any risk of hemorrhage). Once the frenulum has been removed, the male regains his ability or desire to mount and can be used as stud, because no pattern of inheritance has been demonstrated, at least in the dog [98].

An incomplete fusion of the median raphe of the penis, prepuce, or scrotum causes hypospadia, a defect in which the urethral opening is abnormally located ventrally to the tip of the penis (glandular hypospadia), ventral to the body of the penis (penile hypospadia), at the level of the scrotum (scrotal hypospadia), or in the perineal area (perineal hypospadia) (Fig. 13). This is attributable to incomplete masculinization of the urogenital sinus during the process

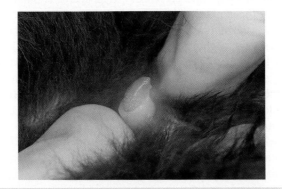

Fig. 12. A persistent frenulum is demonstrated in this tomcat by complete protrusion of the preputium. (*Courtesy of* Antonio Prats, DVM, Barcelona, Spain.)

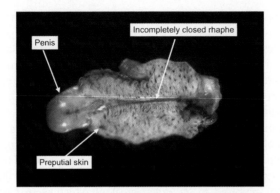

Fig. 13. Failure of closure of the penile urethra and skin leads to a condition called hypospadia. A hypoplastic penis and incompletely closed prepuce of a true hermaphrodite dog are shown. The incompletely closured raphe of the preputial skin extended caudally along ventral midline. The penis was located caudally between the hind legs of the dog, and the urethral opening through which the dog urinated was in the perineal area. A linear opening of the skin extended from the perineum to the penis (tissues shown are approximately 4.5 cm in length).

of male urethral development. The severity of the defect increases from insignificant in the glandular type, which is characterized solely by a slight physical change of urethral opening, to high in the perineal type, which is characterized by a high frequency of other congenital defects, such as cryptorchidism, shortening of the penis, underdevelopment of the glans penis, ventral deviation of the penis, and underdevelopment of the ventral prepuce. Hypospadia is less uncommon than diphallia and persistence of the penile frenulum (70 cases have been reported, of which 24 occurred in Boston Terriers) [101,102], perhaps because it is not only a congenital problem but can be induced by administration of progestins during pregnancy and feeding the pregnant dam with a diet deficient in vitamin A [103]. The presence of hypospadia is often asymptomatic, especially if only the glandular type is present, for which no treatment is necessary. Penile, scrotal, and perineal hypospadias are often characterized by urinary incontinence and inguinal dermatitis because of urine dribbling. Surgical repair of the defect generally requires passing a urinary catheter, dissecting and separating the urethral mucosa from the skin at the mucocutaneous junction, and suturing the incised edges of the urethral mucosa, taking care to avoid placing knots inside the urethral lumen (because this may cause calculus formation). Amputation of the penis and prepuce to the level of the urethral opening is generally performed in case of penile hypospadia, whereas complete penile amputation and scrotal or perineal urethrostomy is required in case of scrotal or perineal hypospadia.

Because of its genetic implications, hypospadia has been proposed as a form of male pseudohermaphroditism (see Table 1) [1,2,56]. Therefore, castration of these animals is always recommended, and breeding individuals with even minor forms of the disease (eg, glandular hypospadia) should be avoided unless other causes, such as steroid administration to the dam during pregnancy, can be confirmed. Hypospadia has been reported in tomcats [4] and is described in cats affected by the testicular feminization syndrome (see section on hermaphroditism) [2].

Penile hypoplasia and penile immaturity indicate underdevelopment of the penis in absolute terms (hypoplasia) or in relation to body weight (immaturity). Penile hypoplasia is reported in intersex and cryptorchid dogs and cats and can be treated by penile amputation and urethrostomy, whereas penile immaturity may be attributable to prepuberal gonadectomy in young animals, and penile atrophy can result from high estrogen levels (because of a Sertoli cell tumor or exogenous administration) in adult animals (reported in dogs) [104,105]. Penile immaturity (smaller diameter, decreased size, and radiodensity of the os penis) and immaturity of the prepuce were observed in dogs gonadectomized at 7 weeks of age when comparing them as young adults (13–15 months of age) with dogs castrated at 7 months of age or left intact [105,106]. Penile hypoplasia was observed in a male tortoiseshell and white cat with one hypoplastic testis, female reproductive organs, and a chimeric chromosomal pattern (38,XX in some cells and 57,XXY in others). Congenital defects of the penis and prepuce in cats are regarded as extremely rare; of 19,646 cats seen at 10 North American veterinary colleges, no such problem was observed in 26 cats with single or multiple congenital defects of the urogenital system [30].

Severe cases of penile immaturity may be characterized by phimosis, urinary incontinence, dysuria, and hematuria and can be treated by surgical shortening of the prepuce and enlargement of the preputial orifice. Less severe cases of penile immaturity not characterized by preputial urine pooling may go undiagnosed. The efficacy of testosterone administration to increase penile size (a common approach for reduced penile size in human beings) is unknown in small animals.

Penile hypoplasia as well as preputial hypoplasia has been observed in intersex and cryptorchid dogs [37,42] but has not been reported in cats. Dogs with preputial hypoplasia are generally presented for protrusion of the penis (owners may erroneously interpret this as a persistent erection problem) or urinary incontinence. Penile protrusion may lead to drying of the penile mucosa, although this occurs more frequently after traumatic loss of the distal prepuce than in congenital preputial hypoplasia, such as incomplete fusion of the ventral prepuce, in which spontaneous healing has been reported by 1 year of age [107]. Surgical reconstruction of the prepuce (by creation of a pedicle extension flap) has been reported to be successful in the dog [108,92].

The inability to protrude the penis from the prepuce, or phimosis, is a defect that can be congenital (in intersex animals) or acquired (because of inflammation, edema, neoplasia, or the presence of scar tissue as a consequence of wound healing after penile or preputial trauma). It was observed in less than 1% of 185 dogs with penile or preputial abnormalities [109]. It has been reported in an adult, domestic short-haired, intact tomcat presented for dysuria, hematuria, and a distended bladder [119]. The differential diagnosis in the cat includes the presence of hair rings [110] and preputial adhesions after prepuberal castration [105,106]. Phimosis can be treated by preputial surgical enlargement, removing a V-shaped piece of tissue at the level of the preputial orifice [104,111,112].

Prolapse of a ring of the distal urethra through the external urethral meatus is reported as a congenital idiopathic problem in young dogs and as a consequence of sexual excitement or urethral infection in adult dogs. The problem is not reported in tomcats. This is a rare condition, of which only eight cases have been observed, six of which were in English Bulldogs [120]. Presenting complaints include penile bleeding and, less commonly, increased urination frequency. Prolapsed urethral tissue generally appears as a classic "red pea" at the tip of the penis, although in one case, the urethral mucosa was observed to prolapse only during erection. The differential diagnosis includes all causes of penile bleeding, such as urethral inflammation, urethral calculi or strictures, fracture of the os penis, and persistent frenulum. In adult dogs, benign prostatic hypertrophy is the most common cause of bleeding from the tip of the penis; therefore, it should be ruled out as a cause of bleeding (but benign prostatic hypertrophy can only occur in postpuberal animals). Induction of an erection can be used to confirm the presence of urethral prolapse but only after a radiograph of the pelvic area has been taken to rule out fracture of the os penis. A conservative approach (eg, isolation from estrous bitches, cage rest, antibiotics, tranquilizers) is generally unrewarding. The treatment of choice is surgical removal of the prolapsed tissue, followed by suturing of the urethral to the penile mucosa. The value of castration in limiting recurrence of the problem is debated; in one case, a dog could be used again as a stud 1 year after surgery, and in another case, the urethral prolapse recurred after 1 year [120].

DIAGNOSTIC AND CLINICAL APPROACH

From a practical point of view, the presence of congenital abnormalities of the reproductive system and other systems should be included in the list of differentials whenever ambiguous external genitalia or incomplete testicular descent is observed in puppies and kittens as well as if the coat color in cats is not in agreement with the sex of the individual or with the coat color pattern of the cat's parents. The clinical approach to diagnose congenital reproductive abnormalities consists of performing a thorough clinical examination of the reproductive organs with a careful inspection of external genitalia, including a vaginal digital examination in female animals and a manual protrusion of the penis from the prepuce as well as palpation of the scrotum (to check for the presence of both testicles) in male animals. The presence of perineal dermatitis caused by urine dribbling should be checked. Further investigation may include (depending on the type of abnormality suspected) other diagnostic imaging tests, such as endoscopic or contrast radiographic studies of internal genitalia (eg, vaginoscopy, contrast vaginography, contrast isterography, contrast urethrography). Contrast radiographic studies should also include the urinary system, because bladder or kidney abnormalities may also be present. Considering coat color in cats may be useful from a practical standpoint, because (1) male cats with a calico or tortoiseshell coat color pattern may have an XXY sex chromosome complement or be chimeras (because the calico and tortoiseshell colors indicate the presence of two X chromosomes) and (2) a queen whose parents' coat color is orange (in one) and nonorange (in the other) should have a calico or tortoiseshell coat; an all-orange or all-nonorange color suggests the presence of an XO sex chromosome complement.

When a congenital problem is suspected, karyotyping should be performed before any other test, because an abnormal result may save time and money otherwise spent in performing expensive examinations. Agreement of the karyotype with the phenotype does not rule out the presence of a congenital problem; for instance, XX true hermaphrodites may present as normal cycling female animals. In such cases, endocrine testing becomes important. Endocrine testing is also helpful in confirming the presence of cryptorchid or ectopic testicle(s) in male animals with the presence of secondary sex characteristics despite the absence of scrotal testes or whenever ambiguous external genitalia may suggest the presence of a congenital disorder. A testosterone stimulation test can be performed in dogs and cats by administering GnRH intravenously at a dose of 25 to 50 µg/kg or hCG at a dose of 50 to 100 IU and assaying serum testosterone before and 1 or 4 hours later, respectively. Values higher than 1.0 ng/mL in the poststimulation sample indicate the presence of testicle(s).

Once the reproductive problem is confirmed, spaying should be considered the treatment of choice, and all removed organs should be submitted for histopathologic examination, asking for serial sections of each questionable sample, including gonads. Ambiguity of external genitalia should prompt clinicians to perform a thorough investigation of the urogenital system of the animal before surgery, including a contrast radiographic study of the urinary system. Congenital malformations of the reproductive system are often associated with congenital malformations of the urinary system. Urinary abnormalities are frequently overlooked in hermaphrodites, but it is well known that they can become a problem later in the life of the patient. Therefore, when performing surgery, it is particularly important to remove all reproductive organs of affected individuals, especially the uterus, cervix, and cranial vagina if present.

Vaginal strictures and septa do not cause any alterations on physical examination; therefore, diagnosis requires an accurate examination of the vagina and vestibule with the aid of diagnostic techniques. Most vaginal strictures and septa are located at the vaginovestibular junction and can be easily detected on vaginal digital examination just cranial to the urethral papilla (palpable in most bitches). If nothing is palpated, one should consider sedating the bitch (if the dog is uncomfortable or is too small to accommodate the finger of the operator) and using an otoscope, a vaginoscope, or an endoscope. If these procedures are not helpful, the next step is contrast vaginography.

Contrast vaginography in the bitch is best performed after withholding food for 24 hours and giving a cleansing enema 2 to 3 hours before the procedure (not strictly necessary). The bitch is then sedated or anesthetized and placed in lateral recumbency. Iodinated contrast medium is diluted with an equal volume of lactated Ringer's solution, a balloon-type (Foley) catheter is filled with the diluted contrast medium and placed into the vagina, and the balloon is inflated at the level of the vestibule. The vulvar lips are held closed with the hand of the operator with atraumatic forceps to prevent backflow of the contrast medium. Infusion of contrast medium is done at a rate of 1 to 5 mL/kg until back-pressure is felt on the syringe or the bitch tries to expel the catheter by contraction of the vaginovestibular muscle. Lateral and ventrodorsal radiographic views should be obtained. The contrast medium passes through the cervix and flows into the uterus only during proestrus, estrus, and the postpartum period. This allows identification of cervical and uterine abnormalities. During contraction of the vestibular musculature, a constriction at the level of the vaginovestibular junction may appear on contrast vaginography. This is a normal phenomenon, which may be avoided by obtaining complete relaxation of the bitch during the procedure. Also, cranial to the urethral papilla, there is an area of vaginal narrowing known as the cingulum, which should not be mistaken for a vaginal stricture.

Vaginal strictures or septa can be treated with digital manipulation (manual dilation under sedation) or removed surgically via an episiotomy. Manual dilation is anecdotally reported from dog breeders as an effective treatment. Recurrence of a vaginal stricture after manual dilation has been observed, however [89]. In a review of 21 cases of canine circumferential vaginal strictures treated manually, 13 showed a poor response and 1 a fair response, whereas the problem did not recur in only 7 (33%) of 21 cases [84]. Small vaginal septa may be broken down using digital manipulation. Larger septa may be excised and removed surgically through an episiotomy by ligation and surgical removal or by electrocauterization. Circumferential vaginal strictures may be treated by resecting the stenotic area or performing a vaginoplasty or vaginectomy [84]. The percentage of successful cases varies, being higher with a vaginectomy than with a vaginoplasty because of postoperative scarring causing recurrence of the stricture with granulomatous tissue. Bitches with minor strictures may be artificially bred, planning a timed caesarean section if parturition does not occur spontaneously (because minor strictures may resolve on their own at whelping).

The importance of spending time and money in establishing a complete diagnosis of any observed deviation from a normal reproductive system should never be underestimated. Some diseases are hereditary, and some others are not, and this may be crucial for a breeder who is willing to select and breed from a potentially defective animal. For instance, without a karyotype, it is not possible to distinguish whether an ovotestis is attributable to a chromosomal (chimera) or gonadal (XX male) sex abnormality; siblings of XX male individuals may carry the trait and may spread the defect across the population, whereas this does not occur for chimeras. Likewise, gonadal histology and endocrine testing should always be performed to discriminate between a malformation with serious hereditary implications and a defect that is attributable to a chance event. For instance, a bitch with clitoral hypertrophy and a 78,XX karyotype may be normal (clitoral hypertrophy may be caused by recent steroid administration) or may be a female pseudohermaphrodite (caused by steroid administration during gestation) or an XX sex-reversed animal. In this case, a testosterone stimulation test is important to establish whether or not testicular tissue is present; a positive result (testosterone elevation) suggests a diagnosis of XX sex reversal, the genetic implications of which are much more serious than those of female pseudohermaphroditism. Gonadal histologic examination is then necessary to distinguish between an XX true hermaphrodite and an XX male.

In dogs, medical treatment of cryptorchid testicles with GnRH or with various LH or testosterone compounds has been reported. Testosterone administration is not effective, perhaps because its action would be required during gubernacular regression and testicular descent into the scrotum. This phase normally occurs during the first 20 to 30 days of life, a time when testicular descent typically has not been checked. Administration of GnRH or LH compounds (including hCG or equine chorionic gonadotropin) has been attempted with varying degrees of success, although a control group was not included in most studies [19,113,114] and spontaneous descent can be observed until 6 months of age [115]. Medical treatment of undescended testicles has serious ethical implications and should be discussed carefully with the owner, because spreading of the genetic base of this defect should be discouraged even if the dog (or cat) is not intended to be used for showing or competing purposes. Whenever cryptorchidism is diagnosed, the presence of other congenital defects (eg, penile or preputial defects; patellar, tarsal, and tail abnormalities; inguinal or umbilical hernia; heart or eye abnormalities) should be checked.

When performing an elective gonadectomy on a purebred pet, care should be taken to evaluate the entire reproductive system, especially if any deviation from normality is suspected based on gross anatomy of gonads. An underdeveloped or ambiguous ovary, which may be overlooked during surgery, might be associated with abnormalities of the reproductive tract that might make ovariohysterectomy a more indicated option than ovariectomy. Also, confirming that a purebred pet is devoid of congenital problems might be important information for the breeder from a selection standpoint. Therefore, any specimen that appears ambiguous after surgical removal should be submitted for histologic examination. This is especially true for gonads, because differentiating hypoplasia from ovotestis or from a retained testicle without epididymis (eg, in case of testicular feminization), for example, is impossible without histology. Hereditary implications of unilateral ovarian hypoplasia, a defect that is compatible with normal fertility [14], may differ from those of a true or pseudohermaphrodite.

References

[1] Meyers-Wallen VN, Patterson DF. Sexual differentiation and inherited disorders of sexual development in the dog. J Reprod Fertil Suppl 1989;39:57–64.

[2] Meyers-Wallen VN, Patterson DF. Disorders of sexual development in dogs and cats. In: Kirk RW, editor. Current veterinary therapy, small animal practice XIII. Philadelphia: WB Saunders; 1989. p. 1261–9.

[3] Johnston SD. Premature gonadal failure in female dogs and cats. J Reprod Fertil Suppl 1989;39:65–72.

[4] Bloom F. Pathology of the dog and cat. Evanston (IL): American Veterinary Publications; 1954.

[5] Reis RH. Unilateral urogenital agenesis with unilateral pregnancy and vascular abnormalities in the cat (Felis domestica). Wasmann Journal of Biology 1966;24:209–22.

[6] Rocken H. Ovarialtumor und ovaraplsie bei einer katze [Ovarian tumor and ovarian aplasia in a queen]. Tierarztl Prax 1983;11:245–7 [in German].

[7] Smith FWK, Buoen LC, Weber AF, et al. X-chromosome monosomy (77,Xo) in a Dobermann pinscher with gonadal dysgenesis. J Vet Intern Med 1989;3:90–5.

[8] Lofstedt RM, Bouen LC, Weber AF, et al. Prolonged proestrus in a bitch with X chromosomal monosomy (77,XO). J Am Vet Med Assoc 1992;200:1104–6.

[9] Johnston SD, Bouen LC, Weber AF, et al. X-trisomy in an Airedale bitch with ovarian dysplasia and primary anoestrus. Theriogenology 1985;24:597–607.

[10] Johnston SD, Bouen LC, Madl JE, et al. X-chromosome monosomy (37,XO) in a Burmese cat with gonadal dysgenesis. J Am Vet Med Assoc 1983;182:986–9.

[11] Long SE, Berepubo NA. A 37,XO complement in a kitten. J Small Anim Pract 1980;21: 627–31.

[12] Manna GK, Sarkar CS. An XO female house cat, Felis catus. Chromosome Info Svc 1988;45:10–2.

[13] Norby DE, Hegreberg GA, Thuline HC, et al. An XO cat. Cytogenet Cell Genet 1974;13: 448–53.

[14] Thomsen PD, Byskov AG, Basse A. Fertility in two cats with X-chromosome mosaicism and unilateral ovarian dysgenesis. J Reprod Fertil 1987;80:43–7.

[15] Stein BS. Tumors of the feline genital tract. J Am Anim Hosp Assoc 1981;17:1022–5.

[16] Anonymous. Third ovary in a cat. Mod Vet Pract 1977;58:199.

[17] Altera KP, Miller LN. Recognition of feline paraovarian nodules as ectopic adrenocortical tissue. J Am Vet Med Assoc 1986;189:71–2.

[18] Baumans V, Dijkstra G, Wensing CJG. The role of a non-androgenic testicular factor in the process of testicular descent in the dog. Int J Androl 1983;6:541–52.

[19] Ravaszova O, Mesaros P, Lukan M, et al. Testicular descent in dogs and therapeutic measures. Problems of abnormal descending testes. Folia Vet 1995;39:45–7.

[20] McEntee K. Scrotum and testis: anatomy and congenital anomalies. In: Reproductive pathology of domestic mammals. San Diego (CA): Academic Press; 1990. p. 224–51.

[21] Bernoulli P. Das Verhalten der Hoden in einigen Missbildungen des Geschlechtsapparates bein Hund [The behavior of testicles in some congenital anomalies of the reproductive system]. Schweiz Arch Tierheilk 1943;85:402–44. [in German].

[22] Latimer HB. Anomalies found in a series of foetal and newborn puppies University of Kansas Scientific Bulletin 1950;33:381. [cited by Bloom F. Testis and epididymis. In: Pathology of the dog and cat. Evanston (IL): American Veterinary Publications Inc.; 1954. p. 213–51.]

[23] Millis DL, Hauptman JG, Johnson CA. Cyrptorchidism and monorchidism in cats: 25 cases (1980–1989). J Am Vet Med Assoc 1992;200:1128–30.

[24] Richardson EF, Mullen H. Cryptorchidism in cats. Compend Contin Educ Pract Vet 1993;15:1342–5.

[25] Romagnoli S. Canine cryptorchidism. Vet Clin North Am Small Anim Pract 1991;21(3): 533–44.

[26] Johnston SD, Root-Kustritz MV, Olson PNS. Diseases of the canine testes and epididymes. In: Canine and feline theriogenology. Philadelphia: WB Saunders; 2001. p. 312–36.

[27] James RW, Heywood R. Age-related variations in the testes and prostate of beagle dogs. Toxicology 1979;12:273–9.

[28] Kawakami E, Tsutsui T, Yamada Y, et al. Cryptorchidism in the dog: occurrence of cryptorchidism and semen quality in the cryptorchid dog. Jpn J Vet Sci 1984;46:303–8.

[29] Ruble RD, Hird DW. Congenital abnormalities in immature dogs from a pet store: 253 cases (1987–1988). J Am Vet Med Assoc 1993;202:633–6.

[30] Priester WA, Glass AG, Waggoner NS. Congenital defects in domesticated animals: general considerations. Am J Vet Res 1970;31:1871–9.

[31] Kersten W, Molenaar GJ, Emmen JMA, et al. Bilateral cryptorchidism in a dog with persistent cranial testis suspensory ligament and inverted gubernacula: report of a case with implications for understanding normal and aberrant testis descent. J Anat 1996;189: 171–6.

[32] Hayes HM Jr, Wilson GP, Pendergrass TW, et al. Canine cryptorchidism and subsequent testicular neoplasia: case-control study with epidemiologic update. Teratology 1985; 32:51.

[33] Mattheeuws D, Comhaire FH. Concentrations of estradiol and testosterone in peripheral and spermatic venous blood in dogs with unilateral cryptorchidism. Domest Anim Endocrinol 1989;6:203–9.

[34] Kawakami E, Tsutsui T, Ogasa A. Peripheral plasma levels of LH, testosterone and estradiol 17-before and after orchiopexy in unilaterally cryptorchid dogs. Jpn J Vet Sci 1990;52: 179–81.

[35] Kawakami E, Hirayama S, Tsutsui T, et al. Pituitary response of cryptorchid dogs to LH-RH analogue before and after sexual maturation. Jpn J Vet Sci 1993;55:147–8.

[36] Henderson W. Cryptorchidism in the adult cat. North American Veterinarian 1951;32: 634–6.

[37] Howard PE, Bjorling DE. The intersexual animal: associated problems. Prob Vet Med 1989;1:74–84.

[38] Diaz JA. Cryptorchidism on a cat. Vet Med 1947;42:159.

[39] Mason KV. Oestral behaviour in a bilaterally cryptorchid cat. Vet Rec 1976;99:296–7.

[40] Memon MA, Ganjam VK, Pavletic MM, et al. Use of human chorionic gonadotropin stimulation test to detect a retained testis in a cat. J Am Vet Med Assoc 1992;201:1602.

[41] Badinand F, Szumowki P, Breton A. Etude morphobiologique et biochimique du sperm du chien cryptorchide. Rec Med Vet 1972;148:655 [in French].

[42] Pendergrass TW, Hayes HM. Cryptorchidism and related defects in dogs: epidemiologic comparison with man. Teratology 1975;12:51–6.

[43] Pearson H, Kelly DF. Testicular torsion in the dog: a review of 13 cases. Vet Rec 1975;97: 200–4.

[44] Naylor RW, Thompson SMR. Intra-abdominal testicular torsion: a report of 2 cases. J Am Anim Hosp Assoc 1979;15:763–6.

[45] Miyabashi T, Miller DS, Cooley AJ. Ultrasonographic appearance of torsion of a testicular seminoma in a cryptorchid dog. J Small Anim Pract 1990;31:401–3.

[46] Heyneman M, Beco L, Heimann M. Intra-abdominal testicular torsion: a case presentation in a unilateral cryptorchid borzoi. Ann Med Vet 1996;140:279–82.

[47] Koch H, Sohns A, Schemmel U, et al. Testicular torsion in an abnormal testis in a pitbull terrier dog. Kleintierpraxis 1997;42:151–2.

[48] Centerwall WR, Bernischke K. An animal model for the XXY Klinefelter's syndrome in man: tortoiseshell and calico male cats. Am J Vet Res 1975;32:1275.

[49] Moran C, Gillics CB, Nicholas F. Fertile male tortoiseshell cats: mosaicism due to gene instability? J Hered 1984;75:397.

[50] Pyle RL, Patterson DF, Hare WCD, et al. XXY sex chromosome constitution in a Himalayan cat with tortoise-shell points. J Hered 1971;62:220.

[51] Thuline HC, Norby DE. Spontaneous occurrence of chromosome abnormality in cats. Science 1961;134:554.

[52] Malouf N, Bernischke K, Hoefnagel D. XX/XY chimerism in a tricolored male cat. Cytogenetics 1967;6:228.

[53] Ishihara T. Cytological studies on tortoiseshell male cats. Cytologia 1956;21:391.

[54] Meyers-Wallen VN, Palmer VL, Acland GM, et al. Sry-negative XX sex reversal in the American cocker spaniel dog. Mol Reprod Dev 1995a;41:300.

[55] Meyers-Wallen VN, Bowman L, Acland GM, et al. Sry-negative XX sex reversal in the German shorthaired pointer dog. J Hered 1995b;86:369.

[56] Meyers-Wallen VN. CVT update: inherited disorders of the reproductive tract in dogs and cats. In: Bonagura JD, editor. Kirk's current veterinary therapy, small animal practice XIII. Philadelphia: WB Saunders; 2000. p. 904–9.

[57] Selden JR, Wachtel SS, Koo GC. Genetic basis of XX male syndrome and XX true hermaphroditism: evidence in the dog. Science 1978;201:644–7.

[58] Walker RG. Hermaphroditism in a bitch. A case report. Vet Rec 1961;73:670–1.

[59] Allen WE, Daker MG, Hancock JL. Three intersexual dogs. Vet Rec 1981;109:468–71.

[60] Randolph JF, Center SA, McEntee M, et al. H-Y antigen-positive XX true bilateral hermaphroditism in a German short-haired pointer. J Am Vet Med Assoc 1988;24:417–20.

[61] Fitzgerald AL, Murphy DA. Bilateral ovotestis in an intersex, mixed breed dog. Lab Anim Sci 1990;40:647–57.

[62] Harman MT. Another case of gynandromorphism. Anat Rec 1917;13:425–35.

[63] Felts JF, Randel MG, Green RW, et al. Hermaphroditism in a cat. J Am Vet Med Assoc 1982;181:925–6.

[64] Curtis EM, Grant RP. Masculinization of female pups by progestogens. J Am Vet Med Assoc 1964;144:395–8.

[65] Jackson DA, Osborne CA, Brasmer TH, et al. Nonneurogenic urinary incontinence in a canine female pseudohermaphrodite. J Am Vet Med Assoc 1978;172:926–30.

[66] Olson PN, Seim HB, Park RD, et al. Female pseudohermaphroditism in three sibling greyhounds. J Am Vet Med Assoc 1989;194:1747–9.

[67] Meyers-Wallen VN, Manganaro TF, Kuroda T, et al. The critical period for Muellerian duct regression in the dog embryo. Biol Reprod 1991;45:626.

[68] Meyers-Wallen VN, Lee MM, Manganaro TF, et al. Muellerian inhibiting substance is present in embryonic testes of dogs with persistent Muellerian duct syndrome. Biol Reprod 1993;48:141.

[69] Hare WCD. Intersexuality in the dog. Can Vet J 1976;17:7–15.

[70] Herron MA, Boehringer BT. Male pseudohermaphroditism in a cat. Feline Pract 1975;4:30–2.

[71] Diegman FG, Loo BJ, Grom PA. Female pseudohermaphroditism in a cat. Feline Pract 1979;8(5):45.

[72] Hare WC. Female pseudohermaphroditism. Feline Pract 1979;9:4–6.

[73] Osborne CA, Johnston GR, Polzin DJ, et al. Redefinition of the feline urologic syndrome: feline lower urinary tract disease with heterogeneous causes. Vet Clin North Am Small Anim Pract 1984;14:409–39.

[74] Peter AT, Markwelder D, Asem EK. Phenotypic feminization in a genetic male dog caused by nonfunctional androgen receptors. Theriogenology 1993;40:1093.

[75] Meyers-Wallen VN, Wilson JD, Griffin JE, et al. Testicular feminization in a cat. J Am Vet Med Assoc 1989;195:631–4.

[76] Sheppard M. Some observations on cat practice (21 cases of uterus unicornis). Vet Rec 1951;63:685–9.

[77] Roberts SJ. Infertility and reproductive diseases in bitches and queens. In: Roberts SJ, editor. Veterinary obstetrics and genital diseases. 3rd edition. Woodstock (VT): SJ Roberts; 1986. p. 709–51.

[78] Schulman ML, Bolton LA. Uterine horn aplasia with complications in 2 mixed breed bitches. J South Afr Vet Assoc 1997;68:150–3.

[79] Robinson GW. Uterus unicornis and unilateral renal agenesis in a cat. J Am Vet Med Assoc 1965;147:516–8.

[80] Johnston SD, Root-Kustritz MV, Olson PNS. Diseases of the feline uterus and uterine tubes (oviducts). In: Canine and feline theriogenology. Philadelphia: WB Saunders; 2001. p. 463–71.

[81] Hare WCD, McFeely RA, Kelly DF. Familial 78,XX male pseudohermaphroditism in 3 dogs. J Reprod Fertil 1974;36:207–10.

[82] McEntee K. Cervix, vagina and vulva. In: Reproductive pathology of domestic mammals. San Diego (CA): Academic Press; 1990. p. 191–214.

[83] Gelberg HB, McEntee K. Cystic rete testis in a cat and fox. Vet Pathol 1983;20:634–6.

[84] McEntee K. Cervix, vagina, vulva. In: Reproductive pathology of domestic mammals. San Diego (CA): Academic Press; 1990. p. 191–23.

[85] Holt PE, Sayle B. Congenital vestibulo-vaginal stenosis in the bitch. J Small Anim Pract 1981;22:67–75.

[86] Wykes PM, Soderberg SF. Congenital abnormalities of the canine vagina and vulva. J Am Anim Hosp Assoc 1983;19:995–1000.

[87] Hawe RS, Loeb WF. Caudal vaginal agenesis and progressive renal disease in a shih tzu. J Am Anim Hosp Assoc 1984;20:123–30.

[88] Meij BP, Voorhout G, Van Oosteron RAA. Agenesis of the vulva in a Maltese dog. J Small Anim Pract 1990;31:457–60.

[89] Root MV, Johnston SD, Johnston GR. Vaginal septa in dogs: 15 cases (1983–1992). J Am Vet Med Assoc 1995;206:56–8.

[90] Kyles AE, Vaden S, Hardie EM, et al. Vestibulo-vaginal stenosis in dogs: 18 cases (1987–1995). J Am Vet Med Assoc 1996;209:1889–93.

[91] Johnston SD, Root-Kustritz MV, Olson PNS. Diseases of the feline vagina, vestibule and vulva. In: Canine and feline theriogenology. Philadelphia: WB Saunders; 2001. p. 472–3.

[92] Dominguez JC, Anel L, Pena FJ, et al. Surgical correction of a canine preputial deformity. Vet Rec 1996;138:496–7.

[93] Potena A, Greco G, Lorizio R. Su di una rarissima difallia in un cane [On a very rare case of dyphallia in a dog]. Acta Med Vet (Napoli) 1974;20:125–33 [in Italian].

[94] Zucker SA, Root MV, Johnston SD. Diphallia and polymelia in a dog. Canine Pract 1993;18:15–9.

[95] Johnston SD, Bailie NC, Hayden DW, et al. Diphallia in a mixed-breed dog with multiple anomalies. Theriogenology 1989;31:1253–60.

[96] Joshua JO. Persistence of the penile frenulum in a dog. Vet Rec 1962;74:1550–1.

[97] Belkin PB. Persistence of the penile frenulum in a dog. Mod Vet Pract 1969;50:80.

[98] Hutchinson JA. Persistence of the penile frenulum in dogs. Can Vet J 1973;14:71.

[99] Ryer KA. Persistence of the penile frenulum in a cocker spaniel. Vet Med Small Anim Clin 1979;74:688.

[100] Balke J. Persistence penile frenulum in a cocker spaniel. Vet Med Small Anim Clin 1981;76:988–90.

[101] Croshaw JE, Brodey RS. Failure of preputial closure in a dog. J Am Vet Med Assoc 1960;136:450–2.

[102] Hayes MH, Wilson GP. Hospital incidence of hypospadias in dogs in North America. Vet Rec 1986;118:605–6.

[103] Ader PL, Hobson HP. Hypospadias: a review of the veterinary literature and a report of three cases. J Am Anim Hosp Assoc 1878;14:721–7.

[104] Proescholdt TA, DeYoung DW, Evans LE. Preputial reconstruction for phimosis and infantile penis. J Am Anim Hosp Assoc 1977;13:725–7.

has a minimal effect in these species. It also occurs during initial suckling through the ingestion of colostrum and lactation, which have more significant effects in these species [1]. This maternal immunity does provide initial protection against many pathogens but, of course, is dependent on the health and immune status of the mother as well as the health of the fetus and neonate. Although this may result in temporary protection for the infant, in the long term, it may be deleterious to that individual's health by essentially keeping that animal naive to different antigens (eg, maternal antibody interference with vaccination of the neonate). Maternal or passive immunization is effective in protecting neonates for the first several weeks of life but begins to decline and lose the ability to protect against diseases rapidly as the maternal antibodies are degraded through natural catabolic processes. Between the ages of 6 and 16 weeks, depending on multiple factors (including the species; amount of maternal antibody produced, transferred, and absorbed; and individual health status of the neonate), most puppies and kittens have maternal antibody levels below protective levels. If present at high enough levels, however, maternal antibodies can interfere with the neonate's ability to respond to vaccination, because the circulating maternal antibody within the puppy or kitten may effectively respond to and neutralize the vaccine antigen or render it ineffective by preventing recognition of the antigen by the immune system [1]. This is one reason for multiple sequential vaccines in kittens less than 12 weeks of age and puppies less than 16 weeks of age. Maternal antibodies can interfere with immunization, although the level of maternal antibody present may not be protective against pathogens.

A functioning immune system is composed of multiple parts. Innate immunity is the oldest (evolutionarily), least specific, and most immediate (in terms of response to potential invaders and/or pathogens) form of immunity. Macrophages, neutrophils, dendritic cells, and natural killer (NK) cells, combined with numerous products produced by these cells, comprise the innate immune system. Examples of some of the chemical components produced and released by these cells in response to microbial invasion include lysozyme, complement, and various cytokines, such as tumor necrosis factor-α and interleukins, as well as various vasoactive molecules, such as histamine [2].

Active immunization is the process of the individual responding to an antigenic stimulus appropriately by natural infection or vaccination. Active immunization is processed through the acquired immune system. The two main types of acquired immunity are cell-mediated immunity and antibody, or humoral, immunity. Cell-mediated immunity is predominantly directed against pathogens that typically are obligate intracellular organisms. Examples include viruses, some obligate intracellular bacteria, some fungi, and protozoa. T lymphocytes are the predominant effector cells and are dependent on foreign protein (antigen) being presented to them before they can take effect against the pathogens; thus, multiple cell types are involved in forming cell-mediated immunity. Antibody or humoral immunity is predominantly directed against pathogens that can survive outside the host or at least survive extracellularly.

Examples include most bacteria, fungi, protozoa, and helminths. Multiple cells act in concert to confer humoral immunity as well, but the primary effector cell is the B lymphocyte [3].

Kittens and puppies have varying degrees of ability to respond to antigens, whether attributable to natural or vaccine exposure, based on antigen load, route of exposure, antigenic virulence, genetics of the individual animal, and levels of persistent maternal immunity. In naive animals whose maternal immunity has declined sufficiently so as not to interfere with an immune response, the first vaccine should stimulate a primary immune response. This initial exposure and recognition process and the ability to produce antibody to respond to the antigen typically take 10 to 14 days. Subsequent exposures to the same antigen elicit a stronger response; a greater amount of antibody is produced, and the subsequent response is faster. This is known as the secondary, or anamnestic, immune response. Although multiple cell lines are involved in this response, subsets of T and B lymphocytes known as memory cells preserve the host's ability to recognize and respond to antigens to which the animal has previously been exposed [2].

DEVELOPING VACCINE GUIDELINES USING RISK ASSESSMENT

To design, recommend, and actuate an effective plan for each patient, a practitioner must have familiarity with multiple variables. Those variables include the duration of protection conferred on the neonate by the mother, the typical length of time maternal antibody may persist and pose interference with the young animal's ability to respond fully to a vaccine, and the length of time needed for an appropriate response. In addition, knowledge of the various diseases that pose risks to pediatric patients and of safe efficacious vaccines available is critical. In essence, we must assess each patient as an individual within the population to provide optimal wellness over the lifetime of each individual as well as the population. This rationale has led to the concept of *core* and *non-core* vaccines, two terms commonly used when discussing vaccination within the veterinary field. Criteria for assigning vaccines into these categories as well as a third category, "generally not recommended," are based on the following factors [4–8]:

1. Morbidity and mortality associated with the specific disease (does the organism cause serious illness, or does it cause a mild transient disease that may pose only minimal risk to the individual or population?)
2. Prevalence or incidence rate of the disease (although a specific disease may not commonly be seen, the organism is ubiquitous in the environment and therefore poses a risk to the individual or population)
3. Risk of the individual for exposure to the disease (eg, indoor-only animal versus free-roaming individual, regional variations of occurrence)
4. Efficacy of the vaccine (does the vaccine prevent infection or simply ameliorate some signs or length of the disease?)

5. Risks associated with administering the vaccine (are the risks associated with that vaccine greater than the risk of the disease?)
6. Potential for zoonotic disease
7. Route of infection or transmissibility

When these criteria are assessed, general guidelines may be generated for the individual practitioner as well as for the veterinary community at large. Again, guidelines are not to be thought of as absolutes, nor are they to be used to establish standard of care. They are, simply stated, tools for each of us to use to promote optimal wellness for our patients when considering all factors affecting the individual's health (environmental, organismal [pathogen and host], owner concerns, and current vaccine technologies) [4–8].

TYPES OF VACCINES

There are multiple vaccines available for our canine and feline patients; yet, most vaccines fall within three basic categories. Assignment of vaccine products (which are considered biologic agents rather than drugs and are therefore assessed and approved by the US Department of Agriculture [USDA] rather than the US Food and Drug Administration [FDA]) into these categories is based on how the product is created. Simply stated, modified-live vaccines (ML) are vaccines created by altering (attenuating) the pathogen in some way so that it is no longer able to cause serious or clinical disease in the targeted species. Modified-live virus vaccines (MLV) are therefore vaccines containing live but avirulent virus. Killed vaccines are vaccines produced by inactivating the pathogen completely, rendering it incapable of reproducing and thereby unable to cause disease. The third category of vaccines consists of recombinant vaccines. There are multiple types of recombinant vaccines, and this category itself has three subcategories. These vaccines use genetic technologies to introduce genetic material directly into the host (no vector is used [eg, purified subunit vaccines, type I recombinant]), alter the genetic material to change its virulence (gene deletion, type II recombinant), or incorporate genetic material from the desired pathogen into an attenuated vector organism (eg, feline recombinant rabies, type III recombinant) [9,10]. Within the near future, multiple new technologies are likely to provide us with even more choices, hopefully providing our patients with better protection against disease with minimal vaccine-associated risks. For a comparison between vaccine types, the reader is referred to Table 1.

GENERAL RECOMMENDATIONS

Vaccines are available in single-dose and multiple-dose (tank) vials. The use of single-dose vial vaccines is highly recommended in these species. Conversely, the use of multiple-dose vials is discouraged because of the increased risk of contamination and the inability to ensure consistent levels of antigen and adjuvant in individual doses from a single vial [4,8]. Multivalent vaccines are not recommended in cats other than the core feline vaccine designed to protect against feline panleukopenia, feline herpesvirus I (FHV-I), and feline calicivirus (FCV). Because of increased inflammation at the site of multivalent vaccines, all other vaccines should be given as a separate vaccine at the indicated site (see discussion on feline core and noncore vaccines) [5,8]. Allowing vaccines to acclimate to room temperature before administration, particularly in cats, is recommended, because the administration of cold vaccines was found to have an increased association with tumorigenesis in cats [11].

The practitioner is advised always to follow manufacturer's directions for dose and route of administration. Using a topical product parenterally or splitting doses should never be done. Administration of a modified-live bacterin vaccine designed for topical administration yet administered parenterally may have serious and potentially fatal consequences (Fig. 1). A full dose is required to stimulate the immune system; there is no medical basis for giving a smaller dose to a toy-breed dog, and this practice could lead to vaccine failure in that animal. If done with a rabies vaccine, the practitioner is not following federal requirements, which carries potential legal implications [4,12].

The interval between various vaccines, whether using the same product serially in the initial series or using different products in an adult animal, should never be less than 2 to 3 weeks. Interference between the first product administered and a second vaccine product may lead to failure to respond to that second vaccine optimally. The exact mechanism of this interference is unknown but may be associated with interferon produced by cells processing an ML agent or by transient immunosuppression by an ML agent. Multiple vaccines administered at the same time do not seem to elicit this interference and is therefore an acceptable practice [6,9]. The reader is referred to Tables 2 and 3 for a comparison between pediatric canine and feline core, noncore, and generally not recommended vaccines.

CORE CANINE PEDIATRIC VACCINES

The diseases that fall within this category carry high rates of morbidity or mortality; they are of public health concern, are readily transmissible, or may be ubiquitous in the environment. In addition, safe efficacious vaccines are available and provide sterile immunity (prevent infection) or confer a high degree of protection (do not prevent infection but may confer protection, such that the animal does not develop clinical signs of disease) [4,5]. Essentially, the vaccines that fall within this category are recommended for each individual within the population regardless of that animal's lifestyle or locale.

Distemper

Canine distemper virus (CDV), an enveloped morbillivirus, has been well controlled because of widespread vaccination programs over the past several decades. The disease still persists, however, and in addition to high virulence, it is readily transmissible. Infection with the virus causes respiratory, gastrointestinal, and neurologic signs and is often fatal [13]. The distemper vaccine is commonly administered as part of a multivalent product. The general recommendation is to use a modified-live or recombinant, multivalent product beginning at 6 to 9 weeks of age and to give serial vaccines every 3 to 4 weeks until

Table 1
Vaccine types, benefits, and associated concerns

Vaccine type	Manufacturing process, method of action	Associated benefits and recommendations	Associated precautions and contraindications
Modified live (attenuated)	Virus or bacteria made less virulent via cell or tissue passage Attenuated viruses able to enter host's cells and replicate Stimulates cell-mediated and humoral immunity	Mimics natural infection Rapid response by host's immune system Many products able to stimulate adequate immune response with a single dose Does not require use of adjuvant Vaccination of a single individual leads to viral shedding, which may be useful in a herd health situation when rapid exposure of multiple animals with an attenuated organism is desired	Potential to cause disease in some individuals (should not use in immune-compromised animals) Potential of organism to revert to more virulent form and cause disease even in healthy animals Special handling of vaccines required (temperature sensitive, shorter shelf life than killed products) Vaccinates shedding the modified-live vaccinal organisms may lead to disease outbreaks in certain environments Parenteral administration of topical modified-live bacterin products may lead to serious disease (eg, abscess at vaccine site, sepsis)

Killed (inactivated)	Virus or bacteria chemically or heat inactivated Organism unable to enter host's cells actively, unable to replicate Stimulates cell-mediated and humoral immunity	No potential to revert to virulence Vaccinates do not shed the pathogen; therefore, no potential to spread through population Indicated for use in immune-compromised animals (eg, FIV+ and FeLV+ cats) Organism does not cause disease in vaccinates Longer shelf life and less sensitive to temperature/handling requirements	Increased lag time of exposure to immune system leading to increased interval from vaccination to protection Because less immunogenic, these products require adjuvants (vaccine virus unable to enter host's immunocytes actively and replicate); products containing adjuvants should be avoided in cats when alternative products with equal efficacy are available Most killed products require a minimum of two doses to stimulate protective response Greater potential for contamination and adverse reactions (require higher antigen load and adjuvants may cause adverse effects)

(continued on next page)

Table 1
(continued)

Vaccine type	Manufacturing process, method of action	Associated benefits and recommendations	Associated precautions and contraindications
Recombinant (subunit, gene deleted, vectored)	Genetic material from pathogen altered in some way; three categories of recombinant vaccine technology use various techniques Subunit vaccines are created by inserting specific genomic regions from the desired pathogen into nonpathogenic bacteria; bacteria then produce protein as coded by the inserted genome; desired protein is then harvested, purified, and used as a vaccine Vectored virus vaccines incorporate immunogenic genomic regions from pathogen into an attenuated non-pathogenic virus	Vector able to penetrate host's cells, delivering genetic material from pathogen into the cell; therefore, no need for adjuvant Rapid onset of immunity Stimulates cell-mediated and humoral immunity No potential for reversion to virulence May be able to overcome maternal antibody interference earlier than modified-live or killed products Does not cause disease in healthy or immune-compromised animals (appropriate for use in FIV+ and FeLV+ cats) Vaccinates do not shed virus	Requires handling similar to modified live products (shorter shelf life, temperature sensitive) Increased cost in manufacturing and therefore increased cost to consumer

Abbreviations: FeLV, feline leukemia virus; FIV, feline immunodeficiency virus.

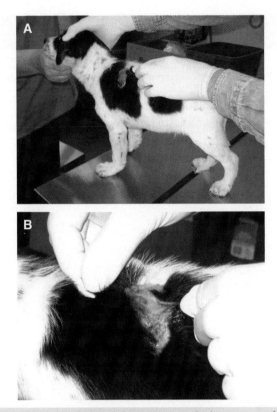

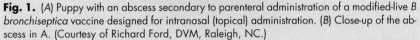

Fig. 1. (A) Puppy with an abscess secondary to parenteral administration of a modified-live *B bronchiseptica* vaccine designed for intranasal (topical) administration. (B) Close-up of the abscess in A. (Courtesy of Richard Ford, DVM, Raleigh, NC.)

the puppy has reached 14 to 16 weeks of age [4,9,14]. Currently, there is one product that contains modified-live distemper virus, canine adenovirus type II (CAV-II), and canine parvovirus (CPV) (Continuum; Intervet, Millsboro, Delaware), but there are numerous vaccines with high safety and efficacy records that also include canine parainfluenza virus. There is also a vaccine that combines a recombinant canarypox-vectored CDV with modified-live adenovirus II, parainfluenza, and parvovirus (Recombitek; Merial Ltd, Duluth, Georgia), and this vaccine seems to be less affected by maternal antibody interference than MLV vaccines [15]. Other studies support the improved ability of recombinant vaccines to overcome maternal antibody interference as compared with MLV vaccines [16,17]. Most puppies receive two or three distemper vaccinations, depending on the age when they are first presented to the veterinarian. It is, however, the interval between or the "timing" of the vaccinations rather than the "number" that is important. Serial vaccinations help to increase the likelihood of a complete response of the patient and thereby decrease the

Table 2
Canine pediatric vaccines: core, noncore, and generally not recommended

Canine	Core	Noncore	Not recommended
CDV	MLV or recombinant beginning at 6–9 weeks, given every 3–4 weeks until ~16 weeks of age		
CAV II	MLV, frequency as for CDV		
Parvovirus	MLV, frequency as for CDV		
Rabies	Killed, single dose, minimum age dependent on state and local regulations (12 or 16 weeks)		
Leptospirosis		Killed bacterin or purified subunit product beginning at 12 weeks, 2 to 3 doses given at 4- week intervals	
Bordetella bronchiseptica		Attenuated bacterin, a single dose of an intranasal vaccine given 1 week before potential exposure (minimum of 4 weeks of age)	
Parainfluenza		MLV, either use topical product combined with B bronchiseptica or parenteral vaccine contained in multivalent DAPP products	
Lyme disease (Borrelia burgdorferi)		Recombinant subunit vaccine (OspA) before exposure to ticks, 2 doses given 4 weeks apart beginning at 9 weeks of age	
Measles			No longer recommended, use recombinant distemper vaccine for high-risk puppies instead of measles

(continued on next page)

| Table 2 | | | |
| (continued) | | | |
Canine	Core	Noncore	Not recommended
Coronavirus			Not recommended
Giardia lamblia			Not recommended
Rattlesnake vaccine			Insufficient data to evaluate efficacy; prevention of exposure, aversion training, and immediate veterinary attention after exposure highly recommended
CAV I			Not recommended; CAV II to prevent CAV I infection is highly recommended

Abbreviations: CAV, canine adenovirus; CDV, canine distemper virus; DAPP, distemper, parvovirus, and parainfluenza; MLV, modified-live virus; OspA, outer surface protein A

risk of vaccine failure that may occur when only one vaccine is administered. In addition, by eliciting a secondary immune response, they may help to increase the level of circulating antibody and decrease the lag time between exposure to an antigen and achievement of maximal antibody level [2]. Potential causes for vaccine failure include an MLV vaccine that was improperly stored and therefore lost its efficacy, the vaccine was improperly administered (wrong route or accidental loss of vaccine onto the skin of the patient), the patient's immune system did not respond (the immune system may have been responding to another antigenic challenge, or the vaccine may have been given too soon after a previous vaccine), and maternal interference [9]. In theory, if a puppy were kept "sequestered" from exposure to this virus, one MLV distemper vaccine administered after 16 weeks of age would confer protection for at least 1 year [1,4]. In reality, however, most pet owners are not inclined to isolate their puppies for the first 4 months of life, nor should they. Early socialization is an important part of families bonding with their puppies. Exposure to various people, other dogs, and new places helps to decrease behavior problems in young adult and mature dogs [18]. As long as the last distemper vaccine is administered after 16 weeks of age, the puppy should be able to mount a strong active response and fully overcome any residual maternal antibody. The current recommendation is to have the puppy return 1 year later (when approximately 16 months old) for administration of another dose of distemper vaccine. After the first "annual" vaccination, triennial immunization is recommended for MLV vaccines [4,19]. Annual revaccination is currently recommended if the recombinant product is used [4,9].

Canine Adenovirus

There are two types of adenovirus that cause disease in our canine patients. Canine adenovirus type I (CAV-I), a nonenveloped virus in the family Adenoviridae, causes the potentially fatal disease infectious canine hepatitis. Clinical signs include fever, depression, vomiting and diarrhea, and potential

Table 3
Feline pediatric vaccines: core, noncore and generally not recommended

Feline	Core	Noncore	Not recommended
Feline herpesvirus FVR	MLV, give 2 to 3 doses of parenteral product beginning at 6 to 9 weeks of age every 3 to 4 weeks until ~12 weeks of age		
Calicivirus	MLV, frequency as for FVR		
Panleukopenia	MLV, frequency as for FVR		
Rabies	Recombinant canarypox-vectored product, single dose at minimum age of 8 weeks of age but varies dependent on state and local regulations		
FeLVª		After viral screening confirming negative viral FeLV status, recombinant canarypox-vectored or killed product, 2 doses given 4 weeks apart as early as 8 weeks of age	
Chlamydiosis (Chlamydophila felis)		In high-risk environments, use parenteral attenuated bacterin product, 2 doses given 4 weeks apart beginning at 9 weeks of age	

Bordetella bronchiseptica	In high-risk environments, topical attenuated bacterin product designed for use in this species, single dose as early as 4 weeks of age	
Feline immunodeficiency virus		Not generally recommended in kittens; viral testing in kittens less than 6 months of age may yield false-positive results because of PMA; vaccination causes positive Ab test
Feline infectious peritonitis		Not recommended; vaccination causes positive Ab test
Giardia lamblia		Not recommended

Abbreviations: Ab, antibody; FeLV, feline leukemia virus; FVR, feline viral rhinotracheitis; MLV, modified-live virus; PMA, persistent maternal antibodies.

^aBecause of increased susceptibility for infection in kittens, vaccination against FeLV is strongly recommended for all kittens. In single-cat households, households with known negative viral status of all cats, and households with indoor only cats, the practitioner may elect to consider this a noncore vaccine.

petechiation and ecchymotic hemorrhage secondary to hepatic dysfunction. In addition, uveitis and renal disease are associated with infection with this virus. CAV-II causes respiratory tract disease. CAV-I is associated with severe potentially fatal disease, and protection against this disease is recommended. Transmission is via the oronasal route and exposure to infected secretions. CAV-II infection typically results in mild self-limiting disease and is therefore considered to be a noncore disease; however, the MLV product designed for prevention of CAV-I has been associated with adverse effects, such as uveitis and corneal edema (an arthus reaction, similar to effects caused by natural infection) [9,13]. The current recommendation is to use the CAV-II MLV because it stimulates the immune system to protect against CAV-I and CAV-II without the associated adverse reaction caused by the type I vaccine [4,14,20]. A modified-live adeno–type II virus is typically included in a multivalent injection (as mentioned previously) and is therefore usually administered at intervals of 3 to 4 weeks, beginning between 6 and 9 weeks of age and ending between 14 and 16 weeks of age. A vaccination 1 year later is recommended before instituting triennial vaccinations.

Canine Parvovirus

CPV is a nonenveloped type 2 parvovirus. The predominant form currently causing infection in the United States is type 2b, but other subtypes exist and cause disease elsewhere [13]. Because the virus is nonenveloped, it may exist (outside a host) under certain environmental conditions and is somewhat resistant to many disinfectants. Transmission is via the fecal-oral route, and clinical signs include lethargy, anorexia, pyrexia, vomiting, and diarrhea (typically hemorrhagic). Young animals seem to be at highest risk for developing severe life-threatening disease. The current recommendation for vaccination is to use a multivalent MLV beginning at 6 to 9 weeks of age and to repeat the vaccine at intervals as stated previously (every 3 to 4 weeks until the puppy is 14 to 16 weeks of age). There has been some concern that certain breeds may be at increased risk for contracting and developing severe parvoviral disease (eg, Doberman Pinschers, Rottweilers), but it is generally agreed that these breeds mount an appropriate response to a quality product if the last vaccine is given between 14 and 16 weeks of age [13,21]. Recent studies using MLV CPV2b strains showed a higher antibody response to CPV2 and CPV2b and that the CPV2b strain vaccines were better able to overcome maternal antibody interference than the CPV2 strain vaccines used [22,23]. An alternative would be to use serial vaccinations of killed virus if the practitioner were concerned about the potential for vaccine-induced clinical disease in one of the breeds believed to be more susceptible to this virus; however, these vaccines are less immunogenic [13]. Immunization 1 year after completing the initial puppy series is recommended, with subsequent triennial vaccinations [4,19,24].

Rabies

Rabies virus, an enveloped virus in the Rhabdoviridae family, is capable of infecting all mammals [13]. Because it is an enveloped virus, it is not stable in the environment and is readily inactivated by most common disinfectants. The virus is transmitted through infected saliva, most commonly from a bite by an infected animal. Clinical signs range from anxiety or other vague behavior changes to pica, dysphagia, photophobia, and paralysis. Because of the zoonotic potential and implications regarding public health, canine vaccination programs are strongly regulated and enforced. The current recommendation is to vaccinate puppies using a killed virus vaccine at a minimum of 12 or 16 weeks of age. State regulations vary as to the minimum age for canine rabies vaccination; in California, the legal minimum age of canine vaccination against rabies is 16 weeks. A second rabies vaccine (killed product) is administered 1 year later and then annually or triennially thereafter depending on local regulations [4,5]. It is the practitioner's professional responsibility to acquire knowledge of and maintain adherence to regional laws regarding rabies vaccination frequency [25].

NONCORE CANINE PEDIATRIC VACCINES

Vaccines in the noncore category have limited efficacy, or the organism causing disease is not readily transmissible or may have limited geographic distribution or prevalence. Additionally, the diseases these vaccines are designed to prevent may be so mild or self-limiting that the risk associated with administering the vaccines may be greater than that of the actual disease. Finally, some vaccines may interfere with common screening methods for disease detection and are therefore not recommended unless absolutely warranted for a specific individual. It is the burden of the practitioner, along with the pet owner, to make decisions regarding which, if any, of the noncore vaccines should be administered to a puppy [4–7].

Leptospirosis

A bacterial pathogen that causes acute hepatic and renal disease, leptospirosis is typically transmitted through urine of infected animals (reservoir hosts include dogs, rats, wildlife, and livestock) and in contaminated water. There are at least two different species (*Leptospira interrogans* and *Leptospira kirschneri*) that can infect dogs, with multiple serovars (variants of the same species) of *L interrogans* causing disease in dogs [26]. Although these organisms have the potential to cause serious disease, dogs are not likely to be at risk in a mostly urban and controlled environment (eg, housed in a fenced yard with no exposure to wildlife or livestock). A dog that frequents rural environments or has exposure to waterways or livestock is definitely at risk of infection, however, and should therefore be protected against the disease. Again, the initial puppy appointments should involve a thorough history and include the owner's plans for that dog's future use. If an owner brings a Labrador Retriever puppy to the veterinarian for "whatever vaccines it needs," it is up to the practitioner to ask: "Will it be a hunting dog, will it be used in field trials, or will it be exposed to wildlife and waterways?" The Border Collie that lives on a working sheep ranch surely should be vaccinated as well. Conversely, a long-haired Miniature

Dachshund that spends its days on its owner's lap is at minimal risk of exposure; therefore, vaccination is most likely not warranted. In essence, the regional distribution, seasonality (increased prevalence during and immediately after the rainy season), and lifestyle of the puppy should factor into the decision as to whether the puppy should be vaccinated. If the decision is made to vaccinate against leptospirosis, the general recommendation is to wait until the puppy is at least 12 weeks of age; at that time, a killed or purified subunit vaccine is administered. Infection is serovar specific, and no cross-protection is seen between different serovars; therefore, vaccination with those serovars known to cause disease in a given region is recommended. Currently, there is one killed purified subunit vaccine (LeptoVax; Fort Dodge Animal Health, Overland Park, Kansas) that contains four serovars (*icterohaemorrhagiae, canicola, pomona,* and *grippotyphosa*); however, the duration of immunity against *grippotyphosa* and *pomona* is unknown, and there are no vaccines available for *autumnalis* or *bratislava*. An initial series of two to three vaccinations should be administered monthly and repeated at least annually thereafter as long as exposure to the agent exists [27]. The recommendation to wait until the puppy is at least 12 weeks old before administering the leptospirosis vaccine is based on the increased potential for adverse events associated with this vaccine and to increase the likelihood of a complete immune response minimizing ineffective vaccinations [4,28].

Bordetella

Bordetella bronchiseptica is a bacterial agent that causes infectious tracheobronchitis. Infection with this agent may occur in concert with other agents infecting the respiratory tract (eg, canine parainfluenza virus, CAV-II). Transmission occurs via direct contact or through aerosolized microdroplets from infected dogs and is most likely to occur under crowded conditions, such as boarding and grooming facilities and dog show venues. The current recommendation is to vaccinate puppies at risk a minimum of 1 week before potential exposure with a combination vaccine containing an avirulent live bacterin for *B bronchiseptica* and a modified-live canine parainfluenza virus. Although the vaccine can be administered to puppies as young as 3 to 4 weeks of age, it is generally not indicated unless the puppy is in a kennel environment [28]. Many organized obedience classes commonly require proof of vaccination against *Bordetella* at the time of enrollment or before beginning the course. The general consensus is that intranasal vaccines are superior to parenteral vaccines because they stimulate rapid local immunity [5,9]. If the puppy is intermittently exposed throughout the year (eg, traveling to shows or boarding or grooming facilities), the vaccine should be administered every 6 months.

Parainfluenza

As stated previously, parainfluenza may occur in concert with other respiratory tract agents. The vaccine recommendations are as stated for *B bronchiseptica* if indicated. There are multiple products available, but the product currently recommended is the combination intranasal vaccine containing a modified-live parainfluenza virus with an attenuated *B bronchiseptica* bacterin. For optimal protection, the vaccine should be administered every 6 months to annually if indicated. Alternatively, many multivalent products containing modified-live CDV, CAV II, CPV, and parainfluenza are available and appropriate for use [9].

Borreliosis

Borrelia burgdorferi is a vector-borne spirochete bacterium responsible for Lyme disease (borreliosis). Transmission occurs when an infected tick (various species within the *Ixodes* genera, also referred to as "hard ticks") bites and remains attached to a host, in this case, a puppy. Direct horizontal transmission is not likely to occur; therefore, the risk to human beings and other pets is thought to be minimal. If a puppy has a significant burden with infected ticks, this, of course, increases the exposure to others in the household; however, because ticks typically do not reattach once they have taken a complete meal, the risk is thought to be quite small unless appropriate tick control is not instituted [29]. Vaccination to protect against Lyme disease is controversial, because the duration of immunity and degree of protection provided by vaccination are unknown and vaccination with some vaccines interferes with standard screening diagnostics [30]. Therefore, vaccination against Lyme disease is warranted only if a puppy is at high risk for tick exposure and only if it lives in a *Borrelia* endemic area. There are killed and recombinant (outer surface protein A [OspA] subunit) vaccines available for use against *B burgdorferi*, and if vaccination is deemed warranted, the current recommendation is to use one of the subunit vaccines before exposure to ticks. The vaccine can be given as early as 9 weeks of age and should be repeated 3 to 4 weeks later [28]. The best prophylaxis is likely achieved by using appropriate tick prevention, such as fipronil with methoprene spray or spot-on products (Frontline Top Spot; Merial Ltd, Iselin, New Jersey), amitraz collars (Preventic collar; Virbac, Fort Worth, Texas), or an imidacloprid/permethrin topical product (Canine Advantix; Bayer Animal Health, Shawnee Mission, Kansas) [30,31]. These products should be chosen and recommended carefully by the veterinarian based on household situations, owner concerns, and age of the puppy.

CANINE PEDIATRIC VACCINES NOT GENERALLY RECOMMENDED

Measles

This virus, also a morbillivirus, can stimulate an immune response that is cross-protective against CDV. The indication for using this vaccine is for puppies that may have maternal antibody to distemper virus sufficient to cause interference with distemper vaccination but not adequate to protect against infection. If indicated (see discussion of special circumstances), a single vaccination with an MLV vaccine should be given intramuscularly as early as 6 weeks of age. Subsequent immunizations with MLV CDV vaccines should be given serially as recommended previously (see section on CDV) [1,4,32]. Canine measles vaccines should never be administered to female puppies older than 12 weeks of age because they may develop an acquired immune response to the virus. This could be problematic if a female puppy vaccinated against measles at 14 weeks of age, for example, later became pregnant. If the dog developed antibodies to the measles virus and maintained immunologic memory, it would confer measles antibody to puppies via passive transfer, thus rendering measles vaccination in those puppies ineffective. A more appropriate alternative to administering a measles vaccine to a young puppy thought to be at risk for infection but too young to receive an MLV CDV vaccine would be to use a recombinant CDV vaccine, thereby decreasing the likelihood of maternal interference [15] (Autumn Davidson, DVM, Davis, CA, personal communication, 2005; regarding the American Animal Hospital Association Canine Vaccine Task Force 2005 guidelines, work in progress).

Canine Coronavirus

An enveloped virus belonging to the family Coronaviridae, this virus is transmitted via the fecal-oral route. Vaccination against this disease is generally not recommended, because the vaccines provide questionable protection and the actual prevalence of the disease is unknown. Those most likely to be infected and develop clinical disease are neonates less than 6 weeks of age. Clinical signs may include diarrhea, possibly hemorrhagic but typically self-limiting. The general recommendation is to vaccinate puppies against CPV (as recommended previously), because this practice seems to confer protection against coronavirus in addition to preventing infection with CPV-2 [4,14].

Giardia lamblia

This protozoal parasite causes diarrhea in canine and feline patients as well as in many other mammalian species, including human beings. Transmission is via the fecal-oral route, with animals contracting the agent from contaminated feces or water. There is a killed vaccine available; however, vaccination against this agent is typically not recommended, because most animals are not at risk to contract the parasite, the vaccine does not prevent infection (it may ameliorate clinical signs and decrease cyst shedding), and the disease is readily amenable to therapy (fenbendazole, albendazole, and metronidazole are off-label uses but commonly accepted as standard of care). Because puppies should be prophylactically dewormed at regular intervals, it is unwarranted to use this vaccine even if the disease is suspected, because a standard anthelmintic dose of fenbendazole given for several days should resolve the infection [4,14,33,34].

Rattlesnake Vaccine

A vaccine designed to protect against envenomation by *Crotalus atrox*, the Western Diamondback rattlesnake, was released onto the market recently. The original provisional licensure was granted to provide possible protection against that single species of snake and was granted for use only in California. Recently, the company was granted extended provisional licensure for multiple states and has extended their claim for potential protection against multiple species of members of the Crotalidae (pit vipers). At this time, no challenge studies have been performed in the canine species to validate efficacy claims; all claims are based on antibody titer to the venom component included in the vaccine, to murid challenge studies, and to anecdotal reports of protection of naturally occurring envenomation [35]. The manufacturer does not claim that vaccination with this product completely protects against the effects of envenomation; rather, the manufacturer claims that it may slow the onset of clinical signs and decrease the severity of signs. Immediate veterinary care is still the "gold standard" for any snakebite. Because of the great potential for variability in envenomation (site of bite on an animal, size of the snake, amount of venom injected into an animal, and species of snake), field observations and anecdotal reports of protection are difficult to substantiate. Challenge studies done under controlled conditions are likely necessary to validate the efficacy of this product. At present, because of the preceding statements, this vaccine is not recommended for general use. Aversion training and keeping dogs out of areas known to favor rattlesnake habitation as well as immediate veterinary evaluation and care are still the standard recommendations for preventing and treating disease associated with rattlesnake envenomation.

Canine Adenovirus Type I
As stated in the canine core vaccine section, CAV-I causes serious disease in dogs; however, the use of the CAV-I vaccine is associated with a high incidence of adverse events. Vaccination with the CAV-II vaccine induces an immune response that is protective against CAV-I and CAV-II without the adverse effects. The recommendation is to use the CAV-II vaccine as part of the canine core vaccination program; the CAV-I vaccine should not be used [4].

CORE FELINE PEDIATRIC VACCINES
Feline Panleukopenia Virus
Feline panleukopenia, a nonenveloped parvovirus closely related to CPV, causes serious and often fatal disease in kittens. Transmission typically occurs from direct contact with infected animals, although in utero infection and fomite transmission also occur. Clinical signs typically include pyrexia, anorexia, lethargy, and vomiting and diarrhea. Kittens may be immunosuppressed subsequent to pancytopenia associated with this viral infection. Kittens infected in utero may exhibit cerebellar disease. Prevention is achieved using MLV vaccines beginning between 6 and 9 weeks of age. The standard recommendation is to use a parenteral product (as opposed to intranasal products, which have a higher incidence of postvaccinal viral shedding and potential for clinical disease induced by the more virulent viruses in these vaccines) [4,5,8,9]. As is the case for canine CDV, CAV, and CPV, the core feline diseases, with the exception of rabies, are typically administered in a multivalent product in a series. There are numerous vaccine products containing feline panleukopenia virus, herpesvirus I, and calicivirus (see additional discussion). The current

recommendation is to choose an MLV nonadjuvanted product from a reputable manufacturer. Vaccines are administered subcutaneously in the right thoracic limb and given every 3 to 4 weeks until the kitten is 12 to 14 weeks of age. Repeat administration is recommended 1 year later before instituting a triennial schedule [4,8,36].

Feline Herpesvirus I

FHV-I, also known as feline viral rhinotracheitis virus, is an enveloped virus causing respiratory tract disease in cats. Clinical signs include sneezing, nasal congestion and discharge, conjunctivitis, and ocular discharge. In addition, kittens may exhibit pyrexia, anorexia, and lethargy along with oral and/or lingual ulcerations and associated hypersalivation. In some cases, ulcerative crusting dermatitis that may mimic other dermatologic disease occurs [37]. The virus typically causes upper respiratory disease, but the lower respiratory tract may become involved, especially in neonates or debilitated animals. Infection with this virus is lifelong, although many cats "recover" and do not show clinical signs. Cats infected with FHV-I may have recurrent "outbreaks," especially in times of stress or if their immunity is otherwise compromised. Cats may persistently shed the virus and act as a source of infection in shelters, catteries, and multiple-cat households. Therefore, prevention before exposure is key in controlling this disease [37,38]. Vaccination with an MLV or recombinant vaccine beginning as early as 6 to 9 weeks of age is recommended. This is commonly administered as part of a multivalent product and is given subcutaneously in the right thoracic limb. The current recommendation is for kittens to receive a second vaccination 4 weeks later. The last vaccine in the series should be given when kittens are at least 12 weeks old. The vaccine should be given 1 year later before beginning the triennial schedule [4,8].

Feline Calicivirus

FCV causes respiratory tract disease in kittens and cats. Because it is a nonenveloped virus, it is more resistant to disinfectants and may therefore persist in the environment. Signs are similar to those associated with FHV-I, but lameness and stomatitis are also commonly seen. Transmission of FHV-I and FCV is through direct contact, exposure to contaminated secretions, aerosolization, and fomites [37,38]. A newer highly virulent strain of FCV was recently identified and carries a high incidence of mortality. Transmission is through direct contact or via fomites. Prior vaccination against FCV does not seem to be protective against this strain, and adult cats seem to be more severely affected than kittens [39,40]. The current recommendation is as previously discussed for panleukopenia and FHV-I: administering an MLV or recombinant virus parenteral vaccine beginning at 6 or 9 weeks of age, with a subsequent dose of vaccine 4 weeks later (last vaccination should be when the kitten is at least 12 weeks old). A booster vaccination should be administered 1 year later and then every 3 years [4,8].

Rabies

As stated previously, rabies virus affects all mammals; in this country, most documented rabies cases in pet animals occur in cats [41]. Because of the significant risk to pets, wildlife, and human beings, vaccination against rabies virus is highly recommended for all kittens and cats, even those kept inside [5,8]. Local requirements vary, but the general recommendation is that all kittens should be vaccinated beginning at 12 weeks of age with the recombinant rabies vaccine designed for use in cats [6]. This product uses gene-splicing technology: reverse transcriptase is applied to rabies viral RNA to create complementary DNA. The segment of rabies virus DNA that codes (a codon) for the immunogenic protein associated with the virus (glycoprotein G) is then spliced from the rabies DNA and inserted into a canarypox virus. The canarypox virus is attenuated and nonpathogenic to mammalian cells and therefore carries no potential to cause disease in this species. Because the vaccine is essentially a modified-live product, the canarypox virus can enter cells, delivering the codon for rabies virus glycoprotein G to its targeted site. Once inside the cell, the canarypox virus is unable to replicate, but the rabies glycoprotein G codon is preserved, leading the host cell to express the glycoprotein on its surface. This stimulates cell-mediated and humoral immune responses. In addition to the benefit of stimulating both types of immunity, the fact that no adjuvant is needed is beneficial [10]. Rabies vaccines should be administered subcutaneously in the right pelvic limb as distally as is reasonably possible; the level of the stifle is acceptable, and areas distal to the tarsus are not appropriate. Currently, there is only a recombinant rabies vaccine approved for use in cats (PUREVAX Feline Rabies vaccine; Merial Ltd, Duluth, Georgia). The current USDA approval and label state that this product should be administered annually. There are multiple killed virus rabies vaccines approved for use in cats, with initial vaccination occurring at 12 weeks of age and a subsequent vaccination 1 year later. These products are highly efficacious but may carry an increased association with the development of fibrosarcoma formation because they contain adjuvants [5,6,8,11,42]. Because regulations vary depending on the state or region, the veterinary practitioner must be familiar with local laws regarding rabies vaccination in this species [25].

NONCORE FELINE PEDIATRIC VACCINES

Feline Leukemia Virus

Feline leukemia virus (FeLV) is a retrovirus affecting cats of any age, but kittens and juvenile cats seem to be most susceptible to infection [43]. Clinical signs are numerous and nonspecific, and they include pyrexia, failure to thrive, and chronic or recurrent respiratory tract and gastrointestinal disease. Infection in kittens occurs via vertical transmission from the queen to the fetus but may also spread horizontally from the queen to the kitten during lactation and grooming. Transmission also occurs through direct and usually prolonged contact with other infected cats from behaviors like grooming and sharing food and water bowls as well as litter boxes. Viral screening using an ELISA test designed to detect antigenemia should be performed on all kittens, even if their owners plan to house them strictly indoors. Because the ELISA test detects antigen, maternal antibody and vaccination do not interfere with test results. Therefore, kittens of any age may be tested [44]. If a kitten is antigen-negative, the current recommendation is to administer a recombinant vaccine on the second visit. A second dose of vaccine should be administered 4 weeks later, followed by vaccination 1 year after administration of the last FeLV vaccine in the kitten [6,8]. The recommended site for administration of any FeLV vaccine is the left pelvic limb as distally as is reasonably possible [8]. Currently, there is only one recombinant FeLV vaccine available (PUREVAX Recombinant Leukemia vaccine; Merial Ltd, Duluth, Georgia). This vaccine is administered with a needle-free high-pressure device that deposits the vaccine in skin, subcutaneous, and muscle tissues (VETJET delivery system, Merial Ltd, Duluth, Georgia, which is manufactured by BIOJECT, Tualatin, Oregon) [45]. There are killed virus vaccines that are efficacious; however, because they contain killed virus, they require an adjuvant to maximize the host's immune response. Because of documented associations between adjuvants and the formation of fibrosarcomas, the use of adjuvants in cats should be avoided when adjuvant-free products with comparable efficacy are available. The most recent findings linking injections of any type with fibrosarcoma formation in this species further support the use of a needle-free system as a viable means of vaccine delivery [6,11,42]. Under the current vaccine guidelines released in 2002 in the American Veterinary Medical Association Council on Biologic and Therapeutic Agents' report on cat and dog vaccines, vaccination against FeLV is only indicated if a kitten or cat is allowed to go outside or if the kitten or cat lives with an FeLV-positive cat. Because kittens are most vulnerable to infection and may have exposure if outdoors and because immunity increases with age, it is rational to vaccinate all kittens against this disease with a repeat vaccination 1 year later. Subsequent to that, if the cat is housed strictly indoors and does not live with an infected (FeLV-positive) cat, additional vaccinations are not indicated [8].

Chlamydiosis

Chlamydophila felis, formerly known as *Chlamydia psittaci*, is a bacterium that causes upper respiratory tract disease in kittens and cats. The most common sign is conjunctivitis, but sneezing and nasal discharge may also be present. Transmission is typically through direct contact with infected cats. Kittens are most commonly affected but usually recover fully with appropriate antibiotic therapy—topical oxytetracycline (ophthalmic ointment) or systemic tetracycline or doxycycline. Vaccination against this agent typically does not prevent infection but may prevent clinical signs of disease. Because the vaccine does not fully prevent infection and carries an association with adverse events that may be greater than the actual disease, routine vaccination of household pets with this product is generally not recommended. It may be of use in some environments in which the risk of infection is high, however, such as shelters or catteries [8,46]. If vaccination is deemed appropriate by the practitioner, an attenuated parenteral vaccine can be given to kittens beginning at 9 weeks of age, with a second dose given 3 to 4 weeks later [47].

Bordetella

This bacterial agent causes respiratory tract disease in cats, and cats affected by stress, poor nutrition, or overcrowding seem to be more susceptible. Although many infected kittens show mild self-limiting disease with signs that include pyrexia, sneezing, and nasal and ocular discharge, bronchopneumonia has been documented. There is a topical modified-live bacterin vaccine designed for use in this species, but it is generally not recommended for routine use. If the practitioner thinks protection against *B bronchiseptica* is warranted based on the kitten's risk of exposure (eg, attends cat shows, goes to a boarding facility), administration of the vaccine designed for use in cats may be considered [8]. A single dose of the ML intranasal vaccine can be given to kittens as young as 4 weeks of age [47]. The product designed for use in dogs should not be used in cats.

FELINE PEDIATRIC VACCINES NOT GENERALLY RECOMMENDED

There are multiple vaccines in addition to those described and recommended previously; however, many of these diseases pose a minimal risk to most of the feline population or the vaccines are minimally efficacious at preventing infection or disease and therefore are generally not recommended. Additional reasons not to use some of these products are vaccine interference with screening tests and adverse events associated with some vaccines.

Feline Immunodeficiency Virus

A retrovirus, feline immunodeficiency virus (FIV) primarily affects cats by compromising their immune system, leaving them vulnerable to opportunistic infections. In addition to immunosuppression, with most of the effect targeted against the cell-mediated (T-cell) immune response, infection with FIV carries an increased risk for development of certain types of neoplasia, with B-cell lymphoma being the most common. Transmission occurs most commonly from breeding and fighting. The virus is not spread through casual contact between housemates not engaging in the behaviors stated previously, nor is it spread through casual encounters between nonbreeding and nonfighting cats outside. Naturally occurring infection of kittens from queens is rare; however, kittens can become FIV antibody–positive via passive transfer from ingestion of colostrum of FIV-positive queens or queens previously vaccinated against FIV [48]. FIV antibody levels acquired from maternal transfer in kittens that are actually negative for FIV virus decline over the first several months of life. The standard screening test for FIV is an ELISA test designed to detect FIV antibody. The ELISA was designed to detect antibody rather than antigen, because infected cats produce high levels of circulating antibody in contrast to low levels of circulating virus [49]. Because kittens may have circulating FIV antibody, although actually being negative for FIV antigen, it is generally not recommended to test kittens less than 6 months of age. If a kitten is tested and a positive result is obtained, the test result should be repeated with a different methodology (Western blot or polymerase chain reaction [PCR]) and should be repeated once the kitten is older than 6 months of age [44]. If a kitten is truly not infected, the maternal antibody wanes by 6 months of age, leading to seroconversion. If, however, a kitten or cat remains seropositive, the recommendation is made to keep the cat indoors only from that point on so as to prevent infection of other cats and to decrease exposure to potential environmental pathogens. FIV-infected cats can live for years; unless otherwise indicated by concurrent disease, euthanasia is generally not indicated for most owned pets. There is a killed FIV vaccine available, but the efficacy of this product is still unknown. There are five known subtypes of FIV virus, and the vaccine has been formulated to protect against subtypes A and D; however, the predominant subtype infecting cats in North America and Europe seems to be subtype B. It is unknown if cross-protection exists between the different subtypes [49]. Because the vaccine elicits a strong antibody response, vaccinated kittens and cats become seropositive on ELISA and Western blot tests, because both tests detect antibody. A PCR test is available but is currently only performed at certain laboratories. Because of the increased technologic needs and increased costs of this test, it is not considered the standard screening test. If done under specific conditions, it can detect virus and therefore may be of benefit in differentiating between cats with viremia (truly infected cats) and kittens or cats with circulating antibody attributable to maternal transfer or vaccination. Because of the nature of transmission of the virus and interference with the standard screening methods for infection, vaccination against FIV is not currently recommended. Keeping cats indoors if possible, neutering all cats going outside, and preventing exposure to stray or feral cats that may be more likely to engage in fighting behaviors remain the gold standards for preventing this disease [48,49].

Feline Infectious Peritonitis

The disease feline infectious peritonitis (FIP) is caused by a member of the Coronaviridae. Feline enteric coronavirus (FECV) and FIP virus are two phenotypes of the same virus. FECV transmission occurs through the fecal-oral route, where it typically infects the intestinal epithelium, but the organism can be transmitted via fomites and persists for long periods in the environment. Most cats infected with FECV do not show clinical signs of disease or may have transient diarrhea; some persistently shed the virus in their feces [50]. FECV can, however, undergo random mutations within a host, creating FIP virus, although the virus does not mutate to this form in most cats and most cats do not develop FIP. The FIP virus enters and replicates within macrophages, where it can then be disseminated throughout the body. Clinical signs are numerous but commonly include weight loss, failure to thrive, diarrhea, pyrexia, and chronic respiratory tract disease. Two main types of the disease exist, the dry (noneffusive) and the wet (effusive) forms. Both are ultimately fatal diseases [51]. Although there is a vaccine available, efficacy and indication for use are believed to be minimal, if at all [51]. The current recommendation is not to use this vaccine based on efficacy concerns and the minimal risk of infection in most kittens and cats. Infection with FECV and mutation with subsequent development of disease occur most commonly in multiple-cat households (five or more), catteries, and shelters. The standard screening test for FIP is a serologic indirect immunofluorescent antibody (IFA) test designed to detect antibody. This test may be of some value, but results need to be interpreted with caution and concomitantly with signalment, clinical signs, and other laboratory data. Prior vaccination against FIP yields positive IFA results, further posing potential complications in routine screening of this disease. In general, kittens are most vulnerable to this disease, with greater than 50% of cats with FIP being less than 2 years of age [50]. Prevention is directed toward decreasing stress in kittens and cats in multiple-cat households and preventing exposure of naive kittens and cats in environments known to have high endemic levels of FECV and at depopulating catteries known to have high prevalence rates of FECV and FIP [50,51]. Because of the complexity of this disease and the limited space and objectives of this discussion, readers are encouraged to review the texts by Greene [52] and Ettinger and Feldman [53] for a more comprehensive review of this disease.

Giardia lamblia

As discussed in the canine section, vaccination with this product does not prevent infection but may decrease fecal shedding of infective cysts. Because vaccination does not prevent infection and the organism is readily treated with fenbendazole or metronidazole, routine use of this product in cats is generally not recommended [8].

ADVERSE EVENTS ASSOCIATED WITH VACCINES

Vaccines are potent biologic agents designed to prevent disease. Any foreign product administered to an animal has the potential to be associated with an unexpected response by that animal. Although vaccines must meet USDA requirements for safety, efficacy, potency, and purity, there still exists the potential for adverse events with products that have met those standards. Veterinarians should always report adverse events related to vaccination to the vaccine manufacturer. Some adverse events are more likely to occur with certain agents, whereas others seem to have an increased rate of occurrence in certain breeds. Still others may be idiosyncratic and are not predictable. The following is offered as a brief overview of some types of adverse events associated with vaccination and to offer suggestions as to how a practitioner might best respond to and prevent those events from recurring.

The reactions seen most commonly are local inflammation at the site of the injection or general malaise, pyrexia, and anorexia for 1 to 2 days after vaccination [12]. Most of these reactions are self-limiting and require nothing more than monitoring by the animal owner. It is appropriate for the practitioner to note any reaction, along with a description of signs exhibited, in the medical record and to offer supportive care if indicated. In some instances, administration of an ML causes transient mild clinical disease. Supportive care and isolation from unvaccinated animals are recommended, because the vaccinated animal showing clinical disease sheds the vaccinal organism and is potentially infectious to other animals [9]. Contact information for vaccine manufacturers, support agencies, and disease-reporting organizations is included in Table 4.

Feline Injection Site Sarcomas

Feline injection site sarcomas, also known as feline vaccine-associated sarcomas or fibrosarcomas, develop secondary to local inflammation of injection sites. There is an increased risk for development of these tumors associated with adjuvants and certain repositol agents, such as long-acting penicillin and corticosteroid injections [42]. Measures to prevent these tumors are aimed at decreasing the local inflammatory response by avoiding the use of adjuvants in this species and administering only those vaccines indicated for the individual animal. Multiple vaccines should not be administered in one site because this may increase the amount of inflammation in that site. Following the recommended sites for injection is strongly recommended (see individual vaccine sections for specific sites) [5,8]. There are specific guidelines as to how a practitioner should proceed if a cat develops a swelling at the site of a vaccination or injection. The practitioner is advised to monitor the patient closely, documenting three-dimensional measurements and temporal association if a mass or swelling develops at the site of a vaccination. The "three-two-one rule" developed by the Feline Vaccine-Associated Sarcoma Task Force should be closely applied. "Three" refers to persistence of the mass for 3 months or longer, "two" refers to a size of 2 cm or greater, and "one" applies if the mass increases in size after 1 month. If any of these criteria are met, the mass should be biopsied using wedge technique or needle biopsy, allowing for complete resection of the biopsy margins in the future and subsequent referral to an oncologist or surgical oncologist if fibrosarcoma is confirmed. Fine needle aspiration is not recommended for evaluation of potential injection site sarcomas [54,55]. Most vaccine manufacturers have programs established to help defray the medical and surgical costs associated with these tumors, and the practitioner is advised always to notify the vaccine manufacturer whenever an adverse event is seen.

Type I Hypersensitivity

Type I hypersensitivity, also known as immediate hypersensitivity and, in some cases, anaphylaxis, is mediated by IgE antibody. The host's immune system may react to anything contained within the vaccine product, including cellular products used for culture, adjuvant, preservative, and the antigen itself, and such a reaction typically occurs within 2 to 3 hours after the administration of a vaccine. In the dog, the most common signs are angioedema (Fig. 2), urticaria, and pruritus, but symptoms may progress to respiratory distress and fulminant vascular collapse (anaphylaxis). In the cat, the acute onset of vomiting and diarrhea with associated hypovolemia and respiratory and vascular shock may be seen [12]. If an animal develops any of these signs within the first several hours after vaccination, it should be presented to the veterinarian immediately for emergency medical care and support. It is not the goal of this review to offer therapies for shock; thus, the reader is referred to emergency veterinary literature for recommended therapies. The point here is to advise the practitioner to proceed with caution when using vaccines that may have a higher incidence of these reactions or in breeds that may be at increased risk for immediate hypersensitivity. The increased association between leptospirosis vaccines and type I reactions is well documented, and there are reports that toy breeds, particularly Miniature Dachshunds, may be at increased risk for type I reactions associated with leptospirosis vaccination [9]. If an animal does have a type I reaction to a vaccine, the signs exhibited by the patient, interval between vaccine administration and onset of signs, and therapeutics administered should be well documented in the medical record as well as plans for future vaccination of that patient. Ideally, once an animal has this type of reaction to a vaccine, that product should not be used again in that patient. All subsequent vaccines should be administered after a complete physical examination, and the vaccine should be given early in the day to allow monitoring of the patient in the hospital for several hours; however, if this is not possible, the patient should remain in the veterinary hospital for monitoring for at least 30 minutes, followed by subsequent monitoring by the owner at home for several hours. Pretreatment with diphenhydramine is an option; it is given parenterally (subcutaneous or intramuscular route) at a dose of 1.0–2.0 mg/kg 15 to 30 minutes before vaccination if hypersensitivity is a concern. Administration of corticosteroids concurrently with vaccination to prevent a hypersensitivity reaction is neither appropriate nor recommended because of potential immunosuppression and vaccine interference, however [9,56]. The patient's medical record should be identified, outside and inside, to prevent future accidental readministration of that product. Advising the owner that the patient should never receive that product again is important.

Type II Hypersensitivity

Type II hypersensitivity reactions (autoimmune reactions) are suspected to occur in dogs secondary to vaccine administration. Although this theory is yet unproven, there are reports of dogs developing immune-mediated thrombocytopenia and immune-mediated hemolytic anemia temporally associated with recent vaccination. If a dog develops either of these conditions within 1 to 2 months after vaccine administration, the practitioner would be advised to consider the risk/benefit ratio of subsequent use of that product in that patient [9,57].

Type III Hypersensitivity

Type III hypersensitivity reactions are immune complex reactions. Examples include the anterior uveitis associated with the use of the CAV-I vaccine and

Table 4
Support organizations, regulatory and disease-reporting agencies, and vaccine manufacturers

Agency or company	Address	Website and telephone number	Support available
American Animal Hospital Association	American Animal Hospital Association 12575 West Bayaud Avenue Lakewood, CO 80228	www.aahanet.org 303.986.2800	Position statements on current vaccination guidelines, standards for care and conduct
American Association of Feline Practitioners	American Association of Feline Practitioners 203 Towne Center Drive Hillsborough, NJ 08844–4693	www.aafponline.org 800.204.3514	Position statements on viral screening, vaccination guidelines
American Veterinary Medical Association	American Veterinary Medical Association 1931 North Meacham Road, Suite 100 Schaumburg, IL 60173–4360	www.avma.org 847.925.8070	Links to available multiple sites; position statements on vaccination guidelines, zoonotic disease prevention, and adverse event reporting (Feline Vaccine Sarcoma Task Force)
Centers for Disease Control	Centers for Disease Control and Prevention 1600 Clifton Road NE, Atlanta, GA 30333	www.cdc.gov 800.311.3435	United States government agency (Department of Health and Human Services), current information regarding infectious and non-infectious diseases
Center for Veterinary Biologics	Center for Veterinary Biologics 510 South 17th Street Suite 104 Ames, IA 50010	www.aphis.usda.gov 800.752.6255	Division of United States Department of Agriculture, contact agency for reporting adverse events associated with veterinary biologics

National Association of State Public Health Veterinarians	National Association of State Public Health Veterinarians	www.nasphv.org	Compendium of Animal Rabies Prevention and Control, rabies vaccination certificates available, list of all state veterinarians available on-line
Bio-Ceutic	Boehringer Ingelheim Animal Health 2621 North Belt Highway St. Joseph, MO 64506	www.boehringer-ingelheim.com Technical services: 800.325.9167	Manufacturer
Delmont Laboratories	Delmont Laboratories 715 Harvard Avenue PO Box 269 Swarthmore, PA 19081	www.delmont.com Technical services: 800.562.5541	Manufacturer
Fort Dodge Animal Health	Fort Dodge Animal Health 9225 Indian Creek Parkway, PO Box 25945 Overland Park, KS 66225	www.wyeth.com Technical services: 800.533.8536	Manufacturer
Heska Corporation	Heska Corporation 3760 Rocky Mountain Avenue, Loveland, CO 80538	www.heska.com Technical services: 888.437.5287	Manufacturer
Intervet	Intervet 29160 Intervet Lane, PO Box 328 Millsboro, DE 19966	www.intervetusa.com Technical services: 800.992.8051	Manufacturer
Merial Ltd	Merial Ltd 3239 Satellite Boulevard Duluth, GA 30096–4640	us.merial.com Technical services: 888.637.4251, ext.3	Manufacturer
Pfizer Animal Health	Pfizer Animal Health Whiteland Business Park 812 Springdale Drive Exton, PA 19341	www.pfizer.com Technical services: 800.366.5288	Manufacturer
Schering-Plough Animal Health Corporation	Schering-Plough Animal Health Corporation 1095 Morris Avenue Union, NJ 07083	www.spah.com Technical services: 800.224.5318	Manufacturer
Virbac Corporation	Virbac Corporation 3200 Meacham Boulevard Ft. Worth, TX 76137	www.virbaccorp.com Technical services: 800.338.3659	Manufacturer

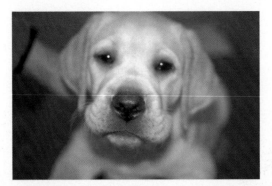

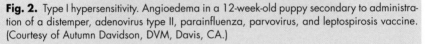

Fig. 2. Type I hypersensitivity. Angioedema in a 12-week-old puppy secondary to administration of a distemper, adenovirus type II, parainfluenza, parvovirus, and leptospirosis vaccine. (Courtesy of Autumn Davidson, DVM, Davis, CA.)

the complement-mediated rabies vaccine–induced vasculitis-dermatitis seen in dogs. Other examples include glomerulonephritis and polyarthritis. Antihistamine administered at the time of vaccine does nothing to prevent the reaction, nor is it recommended to administer corticosteroids concurrently with vaccination. Once an animal has had this type of reaction, subsequent use of that product should be avoided in that patient [9,58].

Type IV Hypersensitivity
Type IV hypersensitivity reactions are cell-mediated responses occurring locally or systemically. Examples include sterile granulomas at the sites of vaccine administration or polyradiculoneuritis. Many sterile granulomas resolve without any intervention; however, for more severe reactions, the practitioner is referred to various medical texts for recommendations [9,57].

SPECIAL CIRCUMSTANCES
The previous discussion applies mainly to puppies and kittens owned by individuals. Puppies and kittens housed in shelters face unique challenges, as do orphaned animals. These animals may not have received colostrum, and it is more likely that their mothers were not adequately vaccinated. The implications are that these animals are less likely to have received maternal antibodies, leaving them more vulnerable in the earliest stages of life. In addition, they frequently are malnourished, have an increased parasite burden, and are placed in crowded environments, possibly with high numbers of endemic pathogens. The American Animal Hospital Association Task Force is currently developing recommendations specifically designed for puppies in these environments. In general, neonates that may not have received colostrum or are housed under these conditions may be vaccinated at an earlier age and ideally should be vaccinated before or at the time of entry into the shelter. The recombinant distemper vaccine could be given in this circumstance and should be administered

every 2 to 3 weeks (Autumn Davidson, DVM, Davis, CA, personal communication, 2005; regarding the American Animal Hospital Association Canine Vaccine Task Force 2005 guidelines, work in progress). Vaccination against additional diseases (canine and feline upper respiratory diseases) is indicated as well (see previous vaccine sections). Husbandry is extremely important in these animals: providing proper nutrition, anthelmintics, and clean and dry housing is paramount. In general, these animals are special subsets of the general population facing challenges that most young animals do not experience. Fiscal considerations and overall population health applies in these cases much more so than to individual client-owned pets.

SUMMARY

Vaccines are perhaps one of the practitioner's greatest tools in preventing disease and maintaining individual and population health. They are to be used with forethought based on the risk of disease to the population and the individual balanced with assessment of the risks associated with individual vaccines. It is the practitioner's role to educate pet owners regarding actual risks associated with undervaccination and overvaccination. The goal is to reach the highest level of overall animal health with the minimum number of adverse events based on scientific and epidemiologic merit.

References

[1] Tizard I. Immunity in the fetus and newborn. In: Veterinary immunology an introduction. 7th edition. Philadelphia: Saunders Elsevier; 2004. p. 221–33.

[2] Tizard I. The defense of the body. In: Veterinary immunology an introduction. 7th edition. Philadelphia: Saunders Elsevier; 2004. p. 1–9.

[3] Tizard I. B cells and their response to antigen. In: Veterinary immunology an introduction. 7th edition. Philadelphia: Saunders Elsevier; 2004. p. 117–32.

[4] Paul MA, Appel M, Barrett R, et al. Report of the American Animal Hospital Association (AAHA) Canine Vaccine Task Force: executive summary and 2003 canine vaccine guidelines and recommendations. J Am Anim Hosp Assoc 2003;39(2):119–31. [erratum: J Am Anim Hosp Assoc 2003;39(3):225].

[5] Klingborg DJ, Hustead DR, Curry-Galvin EA, et al. AVMA Council on Biologic and Therapeutic Agents' report on cat and dog vaccines. J Am Vet Med Assoc 2002;221(10): 1401–7.

[6] Ford RB. Vaccines and vaccinations: guidelines vs. reality. In: Proceedings of the American Board of Veterinary Practitioners, Practitioner's Symposium, Washington, DC, April 29–May 1, 2005.

[7] Ford RB. Vaccines and vaccinations: the strategic issues. Vet Clin North Am Small Anim Pract 2001;31(3):439–53.

[8] Richards J, Rodan I, Elston T, et al. 2000 Report of the American Association of Feline Practitioners and Academy of Feline Medicine Advisory Panel on Feline Vaccines. J Feline Med Surg 2001;3(2):47–72.

[9] Greene CE, Schultz RD. Immunoprophylaxis. In: Greene CE, editor. Infectious diseases of the dog and cat. 3rd edition. St. Louis (MO): Saunders Elsevier; 2006. p. 1073–96.

[10] Tizard I. Vaccines and their production. In: Veterinary immunology an introduction. 7th edition. Philadelphia: Saunders Elsevier; 2004. p. 247–59.

[11] Kass PH, Spangler WL, Hendrick MJ, et al. Multicenter case-control study of risk factors associated with development of vaccine-associated sarcomas in cats. J Am Vet Med Assoc 2003;223(9):1283–92.

[12] Tizard I. The use of vaccines. In: Veterinary immunology an introduction. 7th edition. Philadelphia: Saunders Elsevier; 2004. p. 259–71.

[13] Sellon RK. Canine viral disease. In: Ettinger SJ, Feldman EC, editors. Textbook of veterinary internal medicine, vol. 1. 6th edition. St. Louis (MO): Elsevier Saunders; 2005. p. 646–52.

[14] Greene CE, Ford RB. Canine vaccination. Vet Clin North Am Small Anim Pract 2001;31(3): 473–92.

[15] Pardo MC, Bauman JE, Mackowiak M. Protection of dogs against canine distemper by vaccination with a canarypox virus recombinant expressing canine distemper virus fusion and hemagglutinin glycoproteins. Am J Vet Res 1997;58(8):833–6.

[16] Fischer L, Tronel JP, Pardo-David C, et al. Vaccination of puppies born to immune dams with a canine adenovirus-based vaccine protects against a canine distemper virus challenge. Vaccine 2002;20(29–30):3485–97.

[17] Welter J, Taylor J, Tartaglia J, et al. Vaccination against canine distemper virus infection in infant ferrets with and without maternal antibody protection using recombinant attenuated poxvirus vaccines. J Virol 2000;74(14):6358–67.

[18] Shepherd K. Development of behaviour, social behaviour and communication in dogs. In: Horwitz D, Mills D, Heath S, editors. BSAVA manual of canine and feline behavioural medicine. Quedgeley, Gloucester (United Kingdom): British Small Animal Veterinary Association; 2002. p. 8–20.

[19] Abdelmagid OY, Larson L, Payne L, et al. Evaluation of the efficacy and duration of immunity of a canine combination vaccine against virulent parvovirus, infectious canine hepatitis virus, and distemper virus experimental challenges. Vet Ther 2004;5(3):173–86.

[20] Greene CE. Infectious canine hepatitis and canine acidophil cell hepatitis. In: Infectious diseases of the dog and cat. 3rd edition. St. Louis (MO): Saunders Elsevier; 2006. p. 41–7.

[21] McCaw DL, Hoskins JD. Canine viral enteritis. In: Greene CE, editor. Infectious diseases of the dog and cat. 3rd edition. St. Louis (MO): Saunders Elsevier; 2006. p. 63–73.

[22] Coyne MJ. Seroconversion of puppies to canine parvovirus and canine distemper virus: a comparison of two combination vaccines. J Am Anim Hosp Assoc 2000;36(2):137–42.

[23] Pratelli A, Cavalli A, Martella V, et al. Canine parvovirus (CPV) vaccination: comparison of neutralizing antibody responses in pups after inoculation with CPV2 or CPV2b modified live virus vaccine. Clin Diagn Lab Immunol 2001;8(3):612–5.

[24] Mouzin DE, Lorenzen MJ, Haworth JD, et al. Duration of serologic response to five viral antigens in dogs. J Am Vet Med Assoc 2004;224(1):55–60.

[25] National Association of State Public Health Veterinarians. Compendium of animal rabies prevention and control, 2005. MMWR Recomm Rep 2005;54(RR-3):1–8.

[26] Ward MP, Glickman LT, Guptill LF. Prevalence of and risk factors for leptospirosis among dogs in the United States and Canada: 677 cases (1970–1998). J Am Vet Med Assoc 2002;220(1):53–8.

[27] Langston CE, Heuter KJ. Leptospirosis: a re-emerging zoonotic disease. Vet Clin North Am Small Anim Pract 2003;33(4):791–807.

[28] Ford RB. Canine vaccination. In: Ettinger SJ, Feldman EC, editors. Textbook of veterinary internal medicine, vol. 1. 6th edition. St. Louis (MO): Elsevier Saunders; 2005. p. 604–11.

[29] Greene CE, Straubinger RK. Borreliosis. In: Greene CE, editor. Infectious diseases of the dog and cat. 3rd edition. St. Louis (MO): Saunders Elsevier; 2006. p. 417–35.

[30] Littman MP. Canine borreliosis. Vet Clin North Am Small Anim Pract 2003;33(4):827–62.

[31] Hartmann K, Greene CE. Diseases caused by systemic bacterial infections. In: Ettinger SJ, Feldman EC, editors. Textbook of veterinary internal medicine, vol. 1. 6th edition. St. Louis (MO): Elsevier Saunders; 2005. p. 616–31.

[32] Greene CE, Appel MJ. Canine distemper. In: Greene CE, editor. Infectious diseases of the dog and cat. 3rd edition. St. Louis (MO): Saunders Elsevier; 2006. p. 25–41.

[33] Anderson KA, Brooks AS, Morrison AL, et al. Impact of Giardia vaccination on asymptomatic Giardia infections in dogs at a research facility. Can Vet J 2004;45(11):924–30.

[34] Barr SC. Enteric protozoal infections, giardiasis. In: Greene CE, editor. Infectious diseases of the dog and cat. 3rd edition. St. Louis (MO): Saunders Elsevier; 2006. p. 736–42.

[35] Wallis DM, Wallis JL. Rattlesnake vaccine to prevent envenomation toxicity in dogs. Presented at the Dr. Ross O. Mosier 77th Annual Western Veterinary Conference. Las Vegas, February 20–24, 2005.

[36] Lappin MJ, Andrews J, Simpson D, et al. Use of serologic tests to predict resistance to feline herpesvirus 1, feline calicivirus, and feline parvovirus infection in cats. J Am Vet Med Assoc 2002;220(1):38–42.

[37] Gaskell RM, Dawson S. Other feline viral diseases. In: Ettinger SJ, Feldman EC, editors. Textbook of veterinary internal medicine, vol. 1. 6th edition. St. Louis (MO): Elsevier Saunders; 2005. p. 667–71.

[38] Gaskell RM, Dawson S, Radford A. Feline respiratory disease. In: Greene CE, editor. Infectious diseases of the dog and cat. 3rd edition. St. Louis (MO): Saunders Elsevier; 2006. p. 145–54.

[39] Hurley KF, Sykes JE. Update on feline calicivirus: new trends. Vet Clin North Am Small Anim Pract 2003;33(4):759–72.

[40] Hurley KF, Pesavento PA, Pedersen NC, et al. An outbreak of virulent systemic feline calicivirus disease. J Am Vet Med Assoc 2004;224(2):241–9.

[41] Krebs JW, Mandel EJ, Swerdlow DL, et al. Rabies surveillance in the United States during 2003. J Am Vet Med Assoc 2004;225(12):1837–49.

[42] Kass PH, Barnes WG, Spangler WL, et al. Epidemiologic evidence for a causal relation between vaccination and fibrosarcoma tumorigenesis in cats. J Am Vet Med Assoc 1993;203(3):396–405.

[43] Levy JK, Crawford PC. Feline leukemia virus. In: Ettinger SJ, Feldman EC, editors. Textbook of veterinary internal medicine, vol. 1. 6th edition. St. Louis (MO): Elsevier Saunders; 2005. p. 653–9.

[44] Levy J, Richards J, Edwards D, et al. 2001 Report of the American Association of Feline Practitioners and Academy of Feline Medicine Advisory Panel on Feline Retrovirus Testing and Management. J Feline Med Surg 2003;5(1):3–10.

[45] Grosenbaugh DA, Leard T, Pardo MC, et al. Comparison of the safety and efficacy of a recombinant feline leukemia virus (FeLV) vaccine delivered transdermally and an inactivated FeLV vaccine delivered subcutaneously. Vet Ther 2004;5(4):258–62.

[46] Greene CE. Chlamydial infections. In: Infectious diseases of the dog and cat. 3rd edition. St. Louis (MO): Saunders Elsevier; 2006. p. 245–52.

[47] Richards JR. Feline vaccination. In: Ettinger SJ, Feldman EC, editors. Textbook of veterinary internal medicine, vol. 1. 6th edition. St. Louis (MO): Elsevier Saunders; 2005. p. 612–5.

[48] Sellon RK, Hartmann K. Feline immunodeficiency virus infection. In: Greene CE, editor. Infectious diseases of the dog and cat. 3rd edition. St. Louis (MO): Saunders Elsevier; 2006. p. 131–43.

[49] Hartmann K. Feline immunodeficiency virus infection and related diseases. In: Ettinger SJ, Feldman EC, editors. Textbook of veterinary internal medicine, vol. 1. 6th edition. St. Louis (MO): Elsevier Saunders; 2005. p. 659–62.

[50] Addie D, Jarrett O. Feline coronavirus infections. In: Greene CE, editor. Infectious diseases of the dog and cat. 3rd edition. St. Louis (MO): Saunders Elsevier; 2006. p. 88–102.

[51] Foley JE. Feline infectious peritonitis and feline enteric coronavirus. In: Ettinger SJ, Feldman EC, editors. Textbook of veterinary internal medicine, vol. 1. 6th edition. St. Louis (MO): Elsevier Saunders; 2005. p. 663–6.

[52] Greene CE, editor. Infectious diseases of the dog and cat. 3rd edition. St. Louis (MO): Saunders Elsevier; 2006.

[53] Ettinger SJ, Feldman EC, editors. Textbook of veterinary internal medicine, vol. 1. 6th edition. St. Louis (MO): Elsevier Saunders; 2005.

[54] Morrison WB, Starr RM. Vaccine-Associated Feline Sarcoma Task Force. Vaccine-associated feline sarcomas. J Am Vet Med Assoc 2001;218(5):697–702.

[55] Vaccine-Associated Feline Sarcoma Task Force. The current understanding and management of vaccine-associated sarcomas in cats. J Am Vet Med Assoc 2005;226(11): 1821–42.

[56] Plumb DC. Plumb's veterinary drug handbook. 5th edition. Ames (IA): Blackwell Publishing Professional; 2005. p. 267–9.

[57] Meyer KE. Vaccine-associated adverse events. Vet Clin North Am Small Anim Pract 2001;31(3):493–514.

[58] Tizard I. Immune complexes and type III hypersensitivity. In: Veterinary immunology an introduction. 7th edition. Philadelphia: Saunders Elsevier; 2004. p. 332–42.

Vet Clin Small Anim 36 (2006) 641–655

VETERINARY CLINICS
SMALL ANIMAL PRACTICE

ELSEVIER
SAUNDERS

Pediatric Abdominal Ultrasonography

Tomas W. Baker, MS[a],*, Autumn P. Davidson, DVM, MS[b]

[a]Department of Surgery and Radiological Sciences, School of Veterinary Medicine,
Veterinary Medical Teaching Hospital Small Animal Clinic, University of California at Davis,
1 Shields Avenue, Davis, CA 95616, USA
[b]Department of Medicine and Epidemiology, School of Veterinary Medicine,
Veterinary Medical Teaching Hospital Small Animal Clinic, University of California at Davis,
1 Shields Avenue, Davis, CA 95616, USA

T he use of ultrasound during evaluation of the pediatric patient provides valuable information obtained in a noninvasive fashion with no confirmed adverse biologic effects [1]. Additionally, minimal or no sedation is generally required to complete an abdominal scan. Abdominal ultrasound provides useful data in a short time. The paucity of intra-abdominal fat in pediatric patients results in less informative abdominal radiography but improves ultrasonographic imaging. Acquisition of special equipment for pediatric ultrasonography is usually not necessary; scan heads selected for small animal (especially feline) clinical use are appropriate for most pediatric cases.

EQUIPMENT

Pediatric patients are best evaluated using an ultrasound machine equipped with a curvilinear variable frequency scan head (6.0–8.0 MHz). Many portable machines now have a high-frequency linear scan head (8.0–10.0 MHz) available, which improves quality and also allows evaluation of smaller regional anatomy (eg, thyroid, parathyroid, cryptorchid testes).

PREPARATION

The pediatric patient should be placed in dorsal recumbency within a padded V-trough and gently restrained by assistant(s) holding the forelimbs and hind limbs (Fig. 1). Sedation is rarely required for the basic abdominal scan unless marked pain or apprehension is present. Allowing the patient to become accustomed to this restraint before initiating clipping or scanning usually minimizes struggling and resultant aerophagia.

Clipping the cranioventral abdominal hair using a number 40 blade and wetting the skin with water, tincture of zephiran, or 70% isopropyl alcohol,

*Corresponding author. E-mail address: tbaker@vmth.ucdavis.edu (T.W. Baker).

0195-5616/06/$ – see front matter
doi:10.1016/j.cvsm.2005.12.008

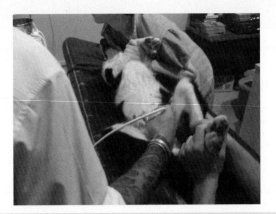

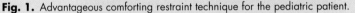

Fig. 1. Advantageous comforting restraint technique for the pediatric patient.

followed by a liberal amount of ultrasound gel, permits the best acoustic coupling of the scan head to the patient, improving the image obtained. Some pediatric patients have scant ventral hair coats and do not require clipping. Care should be taken to avoid excessive chilling of pediatric patients secondary to the application of room temperature liquids followed by evaporation. Electric warming devices (eg, warm water blankets) may cause electronic interference with the ultrasound equipment; warm water bottles or their equivalent are superior [2].

Fasting as much as is safely possible in the pediatric patient minimizes gastric ingesta obscuring imaging of the liver and gastrointestinal gas accumulation interfering with visualization of other abdominal viscera. Preventing urination immediately before the examination permits better evaluation of the urinary bladder.

Serial evaluations can provide useful information when the clinical status of the pediatric patient has changed; clinicopathologic deterioration, progressive lethargy or obtundation, acute pain, changes in abdominal palpation findings, or refractory vomiting or diarrhea warrants repeat evaluation for ultrasonographic signs indicating that intussusception, perforation, or peritonitis has evolved.

NORMAL ABDOMEN

Regardless of the clinical history, the abdomen should be evaluated methodically with the animal in dorsal recumbency. Place the scan head under the xiphoid with the beam in the sagittal plane. Visualization of the liver is achieved by fanning the beam from right to left. The gallbladder is seen on the right; the left liver lobes are seen ventral and sometimes caudal to the stomach. Turning the beam to transverse allows for visualization of the liver between the stomach and gallbladder. This view is good for evaluation of the hepatic border, echogenicity of hepatic parenchyma, and portal architecture. The portal vessels have extremely echogenic walls. Resuming the sagittal plane, scan to the left of the dog past the stomach to the spleen. The spleen is visualized ventrally in the near field. The splenic border, parenchyma, and shape should be evaluated. Following the spleen transversely down the left body wall, you should see the left kidney. Once visualization of the kidney is achieved, turn to the sagittal plane and evaluate the renal border, cortical echogenicity, and pelvic architecture. Dilatation of the renal pelvis is best seen in the transverse plane (Fig. 2). The adrenal is located medial to the cranial pole of the kidney. In the sagittal plane, scan medially to visualize the linear aorta and the renal artery. The left adrenal is located cranial to the left renal artery and caudal to the left cranial mesenteric artery. The left adrenal is visualized as a bilobed structure with the phrenicoabdominal vein at its waist (Fig. 3). With a transverse beam back in the middle of the abdomen, scan caudally to a large hypoechoic structure, the urinary bladder. Evaluate the bladder wall and lumen contents and, dorsal to the bladder, the major vessels (caudal vena cava and aorta). Sublumbar lymph nodes are seen at the aortic bifurcation into the iliac arteries, adjacent to the bladder wall. Sagittal scanning of the urinary bladder caudally allows visualization of the urethra (and prostate in the male animal) (Fig. 4). At the edge of the right ribcage at the renal fossa of the liver, the right kidney is found. The right kidney should be evaluated as was the left kidney (renal border, cortical echogenicity, and pelvic architecture). By scanning sagittally between the right kidney and the caudal vena cava with a fanning technique, the right adrenal is visualized just lateral to the caudal vena cava (Fig. 5). In transverse, find the right kidney and, lateral to the kidney, the duodenum. At the cranial end of the kidney, adjacent to the duodenum, is the right limb of the pancreas. The right pancreatic limb is identified by visualizing the caudal pancreaticoduodenal vein. Turning to the sagittal plane, follow the pancreas, scanning medially to the angle of the body and left limb. The pancreatic body is seen caudal to the stomach and cranial to the splenic vein. The left limb is found caudal to the splenic vein and midline to the cranial pole of

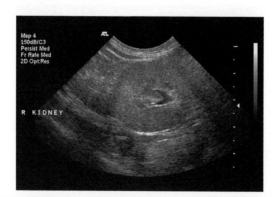

Fig. 2. Renal pelvic dilation (transverse plane).

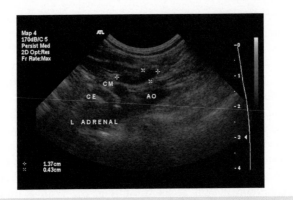

Fig. 3. Left adrenal gland (*cursors*). AO, aorta; CE, celiac artery; CM, cranial mesenteric artery.

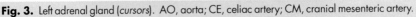

the left kidney. Returning to the transverse plane in the middle abdomen at the mesenteric root, scan for mesenteric lymph nodes and small bowel wall changes. It may take two to three passes to evaluate the entire abdomen in a uniform fashion [3].

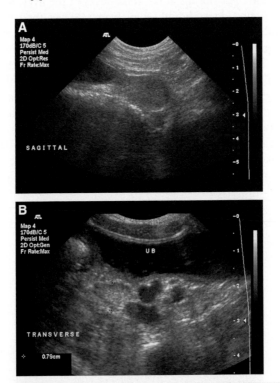

Fig. 4. (*A*) Urethra and prostate (sagittal plane). (*B*) Sublumbar lymph nodes (*cursors*); aortic bifurcation into iliac arteries. UB, urinary bladder.

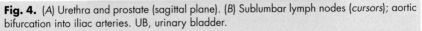

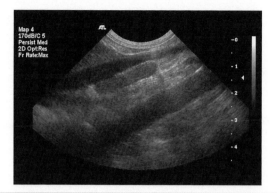

Fig. 5. Right adrenal gland.

COMMON PEDIATRIC DISORDERS

Gastrointestinal Disease

Gastrointestinal signs are a frequent reason for presentation of pediatric patients to a veterinarian. Dietary indiscretion, foreign body ingestion, intestinal parasitism, and infectious (usually bacterial or viral) disease are all common causes for vomiting and diarrhea in the pediatric patient. Physical examination findings, fecal examination for parasites and viral antigens, fecal culture for pathogenic bacteria, and abdominal radiography can all contribute diagnostic information. Abdominal ultrasonography provides additional and complementary information about the presence or absence of fluid in the peritoneal cavity, appearance of gastrointestinal contents, gastrointestinal tract motility, gastrointestinal wall morphology, and mesenteric lymph node appearance and size. Mesenteric lymphadenomegaly is common and not necessarily abnormal in the pediatric patient (Figs. 6 and 7) [4].

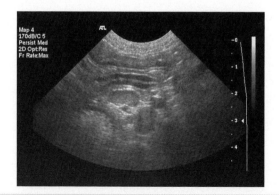

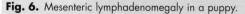

Fig. 6. Mesenteric lymphadenomegaly in a puppy.

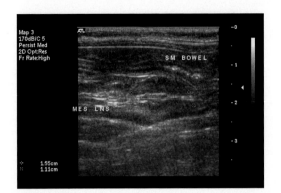

Fig. 7. Mesenteric lymphadenomegaly in a kitten adjacent to the small bowel. MES LNS, mesenteric lymph nodes; SM BOWEL, small bowel.

Gastroenterocolitis

Mild to moderate thickening of the gastrointestinal wall with preservation of wall layering and moderate mesenteric lymphadenomegaly are the most common ultrasonographic findings with nonspecific pediatric gastroenterocolitis, such as that resulting from dietary indiscretion. More severe pathologic findings, such as extensive bowel edema or hemorrhage accompanying infectious gastroenterocolitis, can be associated with changes in fluid volume within the bowel lumen, wall thickening, and loss of normal wall layering. These changes can be regional or diffuse. Fluid distention of the bowel with generalized decreased motility can be seen with functional ileus accompanying gastroenterocolitis (Fig. 8) [4].

Intussusception

Intussusception is not uncommon in young dogs and cats, occurring most frequently at the ileocecocolic junction in dogs and in the jejunum in cats. The

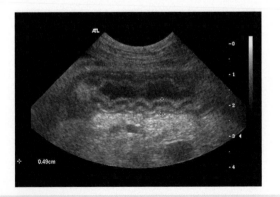

Fig. 8. Fluid-filled small bowel, with cursors measuring full-wall thickness.

classic transverse ultrasonographic appearance of intussusception is a multi-layerd series of concentric rings representing the invaginated bowel wall layers; the outer layer can be edematous (hypoechoic), and the inner layers are more normal in appearance (Figs. 9 and 10) [4]. Discomfort is typically displayed when scan head pressure is placed over the affected area of the bowel. Doppler sonographic evaluation of the bowel and associated mesenteric vessels can provide information about bowel viability [4]. Usually, by the time an intussusception is diagnosed in the pediatric veterinary patient, resection rather than reduction is necessary.

Foreign bodies

Unless radiopaque, gastrointestinal foreign bodies are difficult to confirm radiographically; they are usually suspected clinically based on intraluminal gas and fluid accumulation proximal to the mechanical obstruction caused by their presence. Ultrasonography can provide supportive information and sometimes confirm the diagnosis if the foreign body has a characteristic appearance (eg, ball, trichobezoar, linear foreign body). Typically, a bright interface associated with strong shadowing suggests a foreign body. Fluid peristalsis distal to the object can confirm the suspicion. Balls have a rounded interface with uniform acoustic shadowing. Trichobezoars have irregular bright interfaces and strong shadowing. Linear foreign bodies produce bowel plication recognized as undulation or corrugation of the bowel wall (Fig. 11) [4].

Congenital Gastrointestinal Abnormalities

Pyloric stenosis secondary to hypertrophic gastritis has been reported in a puppy. Focal circumferential thickening of the pylorus primarily involving the muscularis is typical [4].

Enteric duplication or agenesis can be confirmed ultrasonographically in pediatric patients. Duplication is rare and can occur anywhere in the intestinal tract, and the clinical signs may be nonspecific. A fluid-filled juxtaintestinal formation with variable peristalsis and contents can be seen. Enteric agenesis

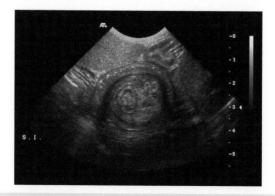

Fig. 9. Intussusception (transverse plane).

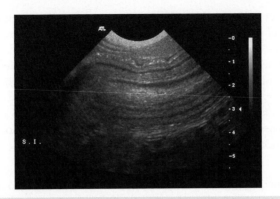

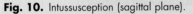

Fig. 10. Intussusception (sagittal plane).

usually results in severe clinical signs in the neonatal period [4]. Ultrasonographic findings usually include marked fluid and gas distention of the bowel proximal to the defect.

Congenital peritoneopericardial diaphragmatic hernias occur in the dog and cat; ultrasonography provides an additional modality for their diagnosis [5]. As with other diaphragmatic hernias, careful evaluation for continuity of the echogenic diaphragm differentiates a true hernia from mirror image artifacts. Evaluation of the pericardial contents can be made using the subcostal (across the liver) or intercostal (using the heart as an acoustic window) approach. Abnormal pericardial contents can include falciform fat, liver, gallbladder, or intestines [5].

Congenital inguinal hernias can similarly be confirmed by ultrasonographic identification of intestines in the subcutaneous space of the affected groin. This can be a dynamic finding. Alternatively, mesenteric fat may be entrapped through the hernia [4].

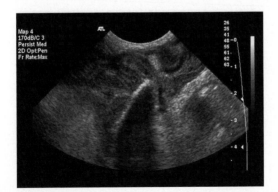

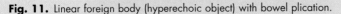

Fig. 11. Linear foreign body (hyperechoic object) with bowel plication.

Congenital hiatal hernias are more difficult to confirm with ultrasound because of the inherent difficulty in imaging the gas-filled stomach and the intermittent nature of the disorder. The stomach wall with characteristic rugal folds can be imaged crossing the diaphragm into the thoracic cavity. Fluoroscopic evaluation can be more informative in these cases [5].

TRAUMATIC DISORDERS

Traumatic diaphragmatic herniation can result in the presence of stomach, liver, spleen, intestines, and falciform fat in the thorax, usually accompanied by effusion of fluid-enhancing imaging. Failure to identify a contiguous diaphragmatic image supports the diagnosis. Positive-contrast peritoneography can be used to confirm the diagnosis if ultrasound findings are not conclusive [5].

Blunt trauma resulting in hemoabdomen is best evaluated with ultrasound. Rupture or crushing trauma to the liver or infarction of the spleen is readily differentiated from normal homogeneous parenchyma. The localization and normal appearance of fluid-filled viscera (eg, bladder, gallbladder) can be reassuring but does not eliminate the possibility of an occult rupture. Serial evaluation is advised, along with the accumulation of clinical data (eg, peritoneal fluid evaluation) [4].

CONGENITAL PORTOSYSTEMIC SHUNTS

Ultrasonography provides a rapid and noninvasive method for screening patients suspected of having congenital portosystemic shunts. Although scintigraphy is considered the most reliable noninvasive method of documenting a portosystemic shunt, its availability is limited to specialty and university practices and its use dictates special handling of the radioactive patient for at least 12 hours. The liver may be small and difficult to image in patients with congenital portosystemic shunts. Imaging the liver from the standard ventral approach can be improved in some cases by using the left ventral intercostal and right dorsal intercostal approaches. The presence of ascites can facilitate the study, as can adding fluid to the stomach and positioning the patient to shift gas away from the scan head and shift abdominal organs caudally. Ultrasound evaluation of portosystemic anomalies can be facilitated by positive-pressure ventilation under anesthesia for the same reason. After surgery, ultrasound can be used to evaluate portal blood flow after surgical banding or coil embolization. Extrahepatic shunts most commonly arise from the portal vein, splenic vein, or left gastric vein in the dog and from the left gastric vein in the cat. Identification of a shunting vessel emptying into the caudal vena cava is difficult but confirmatory. Intrahepatic shunts can be more difficult to identify because of patient size, bowel gas, and liver size. Clipping the hair coat intercostally on the right can allow for transverse vessel stacking (of the aorta, vena cava, and portal vein) and permit visualization of ductal shunts (Fig. 12). There can be right and left shunting of the ductus [6].

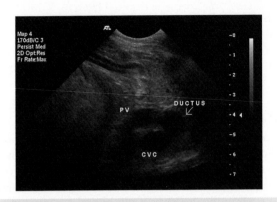

Fig. 12. Intrahepatic portosystemic shunt. CVC, caudal vena cava; PV, portal vein.

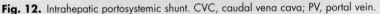

GENITOURINARY DISORDERS

Young dogs and cats are commonly presented to the veterinarian for perceived genitourinary system disorders. Although gastrointestinal disorders account for most acute presentations, perceived urogenital disorders account for many others. Clinical differentiation between the characteristics of normal pediatric housebreaking and immature renal function and true urogenital disease can be challenging.

Renal Agenesis

Congenital renal agenesis resulting in the absence of a kidney can be confirmed with ultrasound. The contralateral kidney typically has normal internal anatomy but is enlarged as a consequence of obligatory hypertrophy. Renal function of the pediatric patient does not equate to that of the adult until 4 to 6 months of age, and compensatory renomegaly may not be apparent until that time [7].

Renal Dysplasia

Until reliable genetic markers are available for the various breed-specific congenital renal dysplasias, ultrasound provides the best method of screening young dogs and cats for these likely heritable disorders. Early ultrasonographic screening is possible in breeds in which morphologic changes are grossly evident (ie, Persian cats, Cairn Terriers, German Shepherd Dogs).

Ectopic Ureter

Congenital ectopic placement of the distal ureter into the urethra, vestibule, or vagina is usually associated with ureteral dilation with or without renal pelvic dilation. Dilation of the ureter improves the sensitivity of the ultrasound study; however, the diagnosis can be elusive. Visualization of a nonvascular fluid-filled structure with a hyperechoic wall passing dorsal to the urinary bladder or obvious insertion of the structure into the proximal urethra suggests the diagnosis. Visualization of the ureteral jets in the bladder suggests normalcy;

however, some ectopic ureters insert initially into the bladder and additionally tunnel distally to terminate in an abnormal site. Visualization of the dilated ureter usually occurs near the urinary bladder (Fig. 13). Visualization of the bladder neck and proximal urethra may be obscured by the pubic bone, making identification of such termination difficult [7,8].

Hydronephrosis can eventually result from an uncorrected ectopic ureter because of flow impedance at the abnormal site of insertion. Urinary tract infection is commonly associated with ectopia because of accompanying urethral sphincter mechanism anomalies; if not detected and treated, it can progress to pyelonephritis and ureteritis. Infection and its associated inflammation in the tract can further alter the ultrasonographic appearance of the kidneys, bladder, ureters, and urethra.

Contrast-enhanced CT is the most sensitive and specific modality for the diagnosis of ectopia; however, like double-contrast radiography, it requires anesthesia, making initial evaluation with ultrasound desirable when ectopia is suspected clinically [7]. The condition is thought to be heritable and is more common in female animals.

Ureterocele

An ureterocele is an uncommon congenital dilation of the ureter near the bladder, appearing as a cystic structure within the bladder lumen or wall. An ureterocele occurs most commonly in association with an ectopic ureter. Diagnosis can be made by scanning the urinary bladder in the transverse plane and watching for strong peristalsis of the adjacent ureter (Figs. 14 and 15) [7].

Urinary Tract Infection

Puppies are frequently presented to the veterinarian because of owner concerns about difficulty in achieving housebreaking and the perception that urination is excessively frequent (pollakiuria). Historical differentiation between a history of true pollakiuria and dysuria associated with cystourethritis and the normal frequency of urination in pediatric dogs with immature renal-concentrating

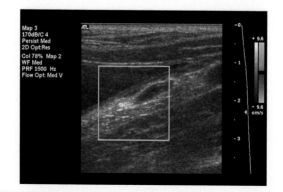

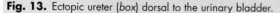

Fig. 13. Ectopic ureter (*box*) dorsal to the urinary bladder.

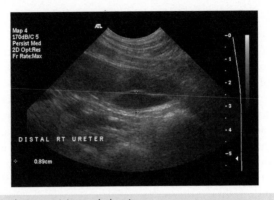

Fig. 14. Ureterocele (*cursors*) (sagittal plane).

abilities can be difficult. A urinalysis and/or urine culture, with urine obtained by ultrasound-guided cystocentesis, can be diagnostic. The bladder can appear normal in acute urinary tract infection. Chronic urinary tract infection can induce bladder wall thickening (greater than 1–2 mm in a fully distended bladder), especially in the cranioventral portion of the bladder. Similarly, early pyelonephritis can have a normal ultrasonographic appearance, and chronic pyelonephritis can produce a dilated renal pelvis, sometimes accompanied by poor corticomedullary definition, increased echogenicity, reduction in renal size, and irregular renal contour (Figs. 16 and 17) [7].

Urolithiasis

Cystic calculi (radiopaque or radiolucent), visualized as discrete hyperechoic focal echogenicities in the dependent portion of the bladder, occur most commonly in pediatric patients with a urinary tract infection (struvite or triple-phosphate uroliths) or portosystemic shunt (ammonium biurate uroliths). The presence of

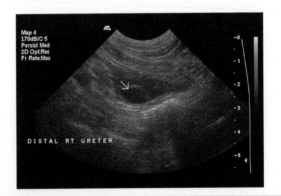

Fig. 15. Ureterocele (*arrow*) (transverse plane).

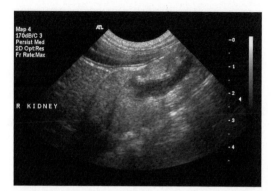

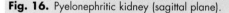

Fig. 16. Pyelonephritic kidney (sagittal plane).

a cystic calculus without a urinary tract infection in the pediatric patient should actually prompt evaluation for developmental hepatic vascular anomalies. Urinary tract infections and cystic calculi are more common in female pediatric patients [4,7].

Patent Urachus

The urachus permits the flow of urine from the bladder into the allantoic sac of the fetus and normally atrophies at birth. A patent urachus in the neonate is characterized clinically by urine dribbling from the umbilicus. The fluid-filled urachus can be identified ultrasonographically, extending cranially from the cranioventral bladder wall. If an incompletely patent urachus is present in the neonate, an urachal diverticulum may result, seen as a divot in the apex of the bladder [7]. Urachal diverticula can predispose the bladder to recurrent infection because of abnormal bladder flow in the region, and surgical excision may be indicated.

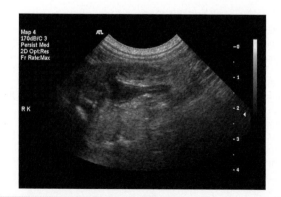

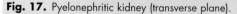

Fig. 17. Pyelonephritic kidney (transverse plane).

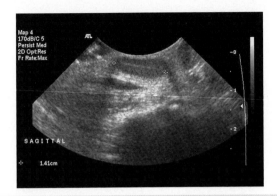

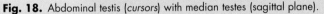

Fig. 18. Abdominal testis (*cursors*) with median testes (sagittal plane).

Cryptorchidism

Ultrasound localization of a cryptorchid testis can confirm the condition in pediatric patients with bilateral involvement whose neutering status is unknown and assist the surgeon in planning the approach (ie, inguinal versus cranial abdominal). The retained testis can be positioned anywhere between the ipsilateral kidney and the scrotum. A systematic evaluation of the region from the caudal renal pole to the inguinal canal can identify an oval homogeneously echogenic structure with a mildly hyperechoic border representing the parietal and visceral tunics. The epididymis is usually distinctly less echoic than the testicular parenchyma, as in the scrotal testis. The cryptorchid testis maintains the anatomic structure, the median testes (a hyperechoic slash), and normal testicular echogenicity despite being reduced in size as compared with a scrotal testis (Fig. 18) [9].

References

[1] Nyland TG, Mattoon JS, Herrgesell EJ, et al. Physical principles, instrumentation, and safety of diagnostic ultrasound. In: Nyland TG, Mattoon JS, et al, editors. Small animal diagnostic ultrasound. 2nd edition. Philadelphia: WB Saunders; 2002. p. 1–18.

[2] Penninck DG. Artifacts. In: Nyland TG, Mattoon JS, editors. Small animal diagnostic ultrasound. 2nd edition. Philadelphia: WB Saunders; 2002. p. 19–29.

[3] Baker TW. Performing the complete abdominal ultrasound evaluation. In: Proceedings of the 2004 Swedish Annual Course in Small Animal Reproduction. Uppsala, Sweden: Uppsala University Press; 2004. p.1–21.

[4] Penninck DG. Gastrointestinal tract. In: Nyland TG, Mattoon JS, editors. Small animal diagnostic ultrasound. 2nd edition. Philadelphia: WB Saunders; 2002. p. 207–30.

[5] Suter PF. Abnormalities of the diaphragm. In: Suter PF, Lord PF, editors. Thoracic radiography: a text atlas of thoracic disease in the dog and cat. Wettswil, Switzerland: P.F. Suter; 1984. p. 179–204.

[6] Nyland TG, Hager DA. Sonography of the liver, gallbladder, and spleen. Vet Clin North Am Small Anim Pract 1985;15:1123–48.

[7] Nyland TG, Mattoon JS, Herrgesell EJ, et al. Urinary tract. In: Nyland TG, Mattoon JS, editors. Small animal diagnostic ultrasound. 2nd edition. Philadelphia: WB Saunders; 2002. p. 158–95.

[8] Lamb CR. Ultrasonography of the ureters. Vet Clin North Am Small Anim Pract 1998;28: 823–48.

[9] Eilts BE, Pechman RD, Hedlund CS. Use of ultrasonography to diagnose Sertoli cell neoplasia and cryptorchidism in a dog. J Am Vet Med Assoc 1988;192:533–4.

Vet Clin Small Anim 36 (2006) 657–666

VETERINARY CLINICS
SMALL ANIMAL PRACTICE

ELSEVIER
SAUNDERS

INDEX

Note: Page numbers of article titles are in **boldface** type.

Changing Your Address?

Make sure your subscription changes too! When you notify us of your new address, you can help make our job easier by including an exact copy of your Clinics label number with your old address (see illustration below.) This number identifies you to our computer system and will speed the processing of your address change. Please be sure this label number accompanies your old address and your corrected address—you can send an old Clinics label with your number on it or just copy it exactly and send it to the address listed below.

We appreciate your help in our attempt to give you continuous coverage. Thank you.

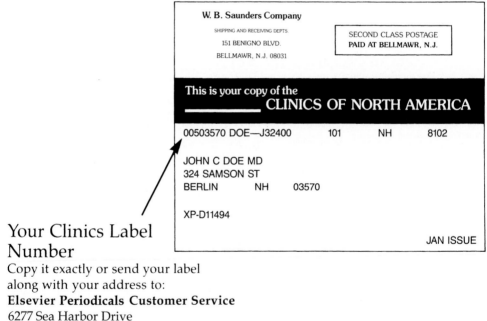

Your Clinics Label Number

Copy it exactly or send your label along with your address to:
Elsevier Periodicals Customer Service
6277 Sea Harbor Drive
Orlando, FL 32887-4800
Call Toll Free 1-800-654-2452

Please allow four to six weeks for delivery of new subscriptions and for processing address changes.